Systemic Therapy in Incarcerated Settings

This book offers both theoretical rationale and practical applications for mental health professionals who seek to implement systemic therapy in correctional contexts.

Delving into the intricacies of systemic therapy and its transformative power in the lives of those affected by the criminal justice system, this book explores how family systems theory and systemic treatment can be utilized with incarcerated individuals and their families. Eman Tadros and expert contributing authors examine the pervasive structural inequalities within correctional settings and offer clinical guidance for working with a range of individuals and unique relationship dynamics, all while considering how to minimize disruption to the individual and their family during the transition from imprisonment to post-release. Chapters explore various treatment modalities within correctional settings including different dimensions of couple and family therapy such as parent-child relationships, reunification, ethics, intimacy, and more. Special considerations are given to working with LGBTQ+ incarcerated individuals and families as well as those from racially and ethnically diverse backgrounds. This book concludes with a call to action and outlines future research directions, encouraging training for therapists and support for justice-impacted families.

This is an essential resource for those who work with incarcerated individuals and their families, such as marriage and family therapists, psychologists, counselors, and clinical social workers, as well as students and researchers interested in family theory and the criminal justice system's impacts on wellbeing.

Eman Tadros, PhD, is an advanced Assistant Professor at Syracuse University in the Human Development and Family Science Department. She is a licensed marriage and family therapist, MBTI certified, an AAMFT approved supervisor, and a Family TEAM leader. She was the former Assistant Editor for the journal *Child: Care, Health and Development*. Her research focuses on incarcerated couples and families as well as dating and romantic relationships. She has published 169 peer-reviewed journal articles and various magazines, blog posts, book chapters, op-eds, and policy briefs.

Family Systems Counseling: Innovations Then and Now

Series Editor: Paul R. Peluso, PhD, Florida Atlantic University

This series is aimed at both current practitioners and students who wish to learn about the historical power and boldness of the family systems approach, but who also need to see it applied to current problem situations. The books in this series will reflect on the pioneering elements of family systems approaches and how they might have been used previously with a particular issue or population.

Intercultural Perspectives on Family Counseling
Edited by Brian S. Canfield

A Family Systems Guide to Infidelity
Helping Couples Understand, Recover From, and Avoid Future Affairs
Paul R. Peluso

An Evidence-Based Systems Approach to School Counseling
Advocating Student-within-Environment
Matthew Lemberger-Truelove and Hannah Bowers Parker

Infidelity
A Practitioner's Guide to Working with Couples in Crisis
Edited by Paul R. Peluso and Taylor J. Irvine

Systemic Therapy in Incarcerated Settings
Clinical Treatment and Applications for Marriage and Family Therapists
Edited by Dr. Eman Tadros

For more information about this series, please visit https://www.routledge.com/Family-Systems-Counseling-Innovations-Then-and-Now/book-series/FSCTN.

Systemic Therapy in Incarcerated Settings

Clinical Treatment and Applications for Marriage and Family Therapists

Edited by Dr. Eman Tadros

Routledge
Taylor & Francis Group
NEW YORK AND LONDON

Designed cover image: Getty Images

First published 2026
by Routledge
605 Third Avenue, New York, NY 10158

and by Routledge
4 Park Square, Milton Park, Abingdon, Oxon, OX14 4RN

Routledge is an imprint of the Taylor & Francis Group, an informa business

ISBN: 9781032894591 (hbk)
ISBN: 9781032882253 (pbk)
ISBN: 9781003542940 (ebk)

DOI: 10.4324/9781003542940

Typeset in Galliard
by codeMantra

Firstly, I dedicate this book to my loving family: My dad who provides, protects and loves. My mom who made education a priority and always said I would write a book. My brother who is both my first student and the smartest person I know. My cousin Christina who has a heart of gold and has been by my side throughout every single one of life's journeys. Secondly, I dedicate this book to all of those carrying the weight of loving someone behind bars, may this book be a reminder that your love, hope, and resilience matter.

Contents

Contributors

Hibba Ahmed recently graduated with her bachelor's degree from the Department of Sociology Criminology at the University of Utah.

Melanie Barbini is a MD/PhD candidate at the University of Massachusetts Chan Medical School.

Katherine A. Durante, PhD, is an Assistant Professor in the Department of Sociology Criminology at the University of Utah.

Eunice Gomez has master's degree in Higher Education Leadership from Northeastern Illinois University.

Yenitza Z. Guzman is an Assistant Professor of Counseling and Higher Education at Northern Illinois University.

Kevin T. Long is a current student in the Mental Health Counseling master's program at the College of New Jersey.

Maxine Notice, PhD, is an Assistant Professor in the Department of Marriage and Family Therapy at Abilene Christian University.

Shannon Pedersen recently graduated with her master's degree in Clinical Mental Health Counseling at Adler University.

Jeffrey Shewell is a current student in the Marriage and Family Therapy master's program at Syracuse University.

Annemarie Sohn is a PhD candidate in the Department of Human Development and Family Science at Syracuse University.

Eman Tadros, PhD, is an Assistant Professor in the Department of Human Development and Family Science at Syracuse University.

Brooke M. Tindall recently graduated with her master's degree in Marriage and Family Therapy from Syracuse University.

Anna Katherine Waters recently graduated with her master's degree in Marriage and Family Therapy from Syracuse University.

Shawn Wunderlich, PhD, is an Assistant Professor of Clinical Mental Health Counseling at Adler University.

Jixuan Zhao is a PhD candidate in the Department of Human Development and Family Science at Syracuse University.

Series Preface

Family Systems Theory or Systemic Family Therapy (and everything that had followed from it) was based on a "crazy" idea. No, literally, it was. In the 1950s Murray Bowen and his team attempted to work with the one condition that neither the Freudian Psychoanalysts or the Skinnerian Behaviorists were able to effect any change: schizophrenia. He decided that the disease was formed and maintained within the emotional processes (or "system") of the family, and that only by changing the family system could the individual patient's schizophrenic symptoms (delusions, hallucinations, etc.) be abated. THAT was the crazy idea, and it sparked a movement that revolutionized the way that children, couples, and even individuals (to say nothing of families) were treated.

One of the guiding forces for Bowen (and subsequently other practitioners) was the work of Gregory Bateson in General Systems Theory. Ideas like feedback and homeostasis took practitioners away from the focus on strict, linear "cause and effect," and instead ushered into the practice of psychotherapy and counseling the idea of circular causality where each member of the system impacts other members (and vice versa). The search for a person to "blame" for a family's problems was replaced with an exploration of system-wide communication, disrupting problematic interactions, and creating collaborative solutions that required everyone's cooperation.

The methods that these early pioneers would employ were equally as radical. Some would do literally anything to disrupt a family's dysfunctional processes and try to effect change. From Salvador Minuchin watching families with anorexia eating meals together, to Carl Whitiker pretending to fall asleep while couples bickered, to the Milan group calling families in-between sessions and giving homework "rituals" for families to complete, to Jay Haley prescribing "ordeals" for clients, or to Virginia Satir physically moving family members around to communicate more clearly, or experience a perspective change; these were all radical uses of systems theory to help families in pain.

These clinicians were creative, courageous, and, at times, counter-intuitive. And while some of their practices might seem odd, outlandish, or even borderline unethical to us today, the underlying principle was to disrupt the family's unhealthy systemic functioning and replace it with a healthier systemic functioning. They wanted everyone to change altogether, not just make individual change. They recognized that this required a boldness, and a commitment to the principles of systems theory that underlie all couples and family therapies today.

However, today many practicing couples and family therapists do not fully understand or embrace the systemic approach that gave family therapy it's power. This is in part due to the rise of the cognitive-behavioral approach, which emphasized individual thought over systemic communication. Related to this, the rise of the evidence-based movement made studying systemic change more difficult than individual change (which CBT was able to do well). Lastly, there was the rise of "managed care," which changed the way practitioners were paid by insurance companies by emphasizing limits on individual sessions (and virtually eliminating reimbursement for family therapy sessions). These movements, taken together over the last 25 years, have drastically changed the training of couples and family therapists as well as the practice of couples and family therapy. It has taken away much of the original systems-focus (and thus the power) of family therapy approaches. At the same time, many private practitioners and agency providers find that they frequently have situations that call for them to provide family therapy, couples counseling, or some type of consultation for parenting or relational issues. Often they have to "wing it" and try to apply individual therapy models to family systems work; however, this is ultimately frustrating to clinicians and leads to poor outcomes for clients.

This series is aimed at both current practitioners and students who wish to learn about the historical power and boldness of the family systems approach, but who also need to see it applied to current problem situations. The books in this series will, where possible, reflect on the pioneering elements of family systems approaches and how they might have been used previously with a particular issue or population. Where some of the historical approaches might be unacceptable to today's standards, authors will be asked to provide a contextually based discussion of relevant issues from all sides (in favor of, and opposed to) of the approach, in the hopes of synthesizing a dialectical solution that reflects the original intent of systemic change.

Acknowledgments

I would like to acknowledge every single contributor and assistant that has helped with this book. I would like to thank all of the wonderful people at Routledge who assisted in the publication of this text. I would like to thank Paul Peluso who invited me to write this book and created the series in which this book is housed. Lastly, I want to acknowledge those impacted by the criminal justice system who show resilience and strength every day.

Chapter 1

Introduction to Incarceration in the United States

Melanie Barbini and Eman Tadros

Incarceration in the United States

The U.S. continues to have the highest rate of incarceration in the entire world (Gur-Arie, 2022). Despite having only 5% of the world's total population in 2014, 25% of the world's incarcerated population was within the U.S. (Collier, 2014). In 2022, the U.S. Department of Justice reported that 1,230,100 people were held in state or federal prisons. This represented a 2% increase compared to the number incarcerated at the end of 2021, but a 41% decrease compared to 2019, when 2,086,600 people were incarcerated (Carson & Klucknow, 2023). For the first time since 2013, prison populations grew in multiple states, with nine increasing by over 1,000 people (Carson & Klucknow, 2023). Females accounted for 7% of the total state and federal prison population, a 5% increase from 2021 (Carson & Klucknow, 2023).

Incarcerated individuals often face compounded vulnerabilities: unstable living situations, limited education, economic insecurity, and high rates of substance use and mental illness. An estimated 10–20% have a serious mental illness, far exceeding community prevalence (Fazel et al., 2016). Prisons are oftentimes a violent, harsh, and psychologically damaging environment where violence and exploitation exacerbate the physical and mental health of incarcerated individuals (*Substance Abuse Treatment: For Adults in the Criminal Justice System: 9 Treatment Issues Specific to Prisons*, 2005). For women, the burden is especially severe; studies show 86% experienced sexual assault, 32% had serious mental illness, and 82% met criteria for substance dependence (Swavola & Subramanian, 2016).

One of the most psychologically damaging correctional practices is solitary confinement: confinement in a 60–80 square feet cell with no human interaction (Cloud et al., 2015). While intended for safety or discipline, most placements are for minor infractions (Cloud et al., 2015). Between 5 and 15% of incarcerated people experience solitary confinement during their sentence (Reiter et al., 2020). Framing solitary confinement as a pressing

DOI: 10.4324/9781003542940-1

public and mental health concern rather than a routine management and punishment measure allows for a more effective dialogue in establishing clinical implications.

Trends in Prison and Jail Populations

There are three main institutions in the penal system: state prisons (long-term felony sentences), federal prisons (federal crimes and pretrial detainees), and local jails (short-term holds and pretrial detention) (Travis & Redburn, 2014). Four broad offense categories lead to incarceration: violent offenses, property offenses, drug offenses, and public order offenses (Carson & Klucknow, 2023). State prisons hold about 87% of incarcerated people while federal prisons hold about 13% (Carson & Klucknow, 2023). In state prisons, roughly two-thirds of individuals are incarcerated for violent crimes, while property and drug offenses each account for about 13%, and public order offenses for 11% (Carson & Klucknow, 2023). Females in state prisons are more likely to be convicted for drug possession while males are more often convicted of violent offenses (Carson & Klucknow, 2023). Contrastingly, in federal prisons, nearly half of individuals are serving sentences for drug offenses, about 43% for public order offenses, and less than 8% of cases for violent offenses (Carson & Klucknow, 2023). Interestingly, females in federal custody are disproportionately incarcerated for drug crimes, about 65% compared to 45% of men (Carson & Klucknow, 2023). Persons held under U.S. military jurisdiction, while small in number, are notable for the prevalence of sexual offenses: about 75% were sentenced for sexual crimes, with more than half for violent sexual offenses (Carson & Klucknow, 2023).

Variation in Incarceration Rates Among Geographic Regions

In 42 states, more than half of the persons in prison by the end of 2021 were serving for a violent offense, with Alaska and California exceeding 80% (Carson & Klucknow, 2023). When the severity of a punishment is determined, the location of the committed crime may be as important as the crime itself. For example, death penalty-eligible cases in Baltimore County were 23 times more likely to result in a death sentence than in a neighboring jurisdiction, and drug arrests in California's King County were 35 times more likely to lead to prison than in Contra Costa County (Mooney et al., 2019). Geographic disparities in the outcomes of similar cases are well documented, including variation across counties under the same state laws (Mooney et al., 2019; Shannon et al., 2017).

Regional differences extend to overall imprisonment rates. The states with the highest imprisonment rates by the end of 2022 were all in the

Southern region (386 per 100,000), with Mississippi (661 per 100,000) leading the nation (Carson & Klucknow, 2023). Other regions had fewer rates: the West (300 per 100,000), the Midwest (288 per 100,000), and the Northeast (148 per 100,000) (Carson & Klucknow, 2023). These imprisonment rates are striking, as states allocate significant money to incarcerate people. For example, Illinois spends an estimated $22,000 in operational expenses to incarcerate one person for a year, and the Illinois Department of Corrections (IDOC) has about $1.5 billion dollars of spending money to allocate for the operation of prison facilities (Harrison et al., 2020; *Illinois State Commission on Criminal Justice and Sentencing Reform*, 2016).

Moreover, the admissions to state prisons increased by 12% from 2021 to 2022 and 17 states had at least 1,000 more admissions to prisons in 2022 compared to the previous year (Carson & Klucknow, 2023). In 2022, compared to the previous year, states released 1% more (Carson & Klucknow, 2023). As the population of state prisons continues to fluctuate, it is important to note that overcrowding remains a persistent problem. Seventeen states had prison populations at or above their lowest capacity measure, and several exceeded their highest design capacity (Carson & Klucknow, 2023). Overcrowding as a direct health consequence: during the COVID-19 pandemic, prisons operating above 100% design capacity had three to five times higher incidence of infection (Leibowitz et al., 2021). The health risks extend beyond prison walls, affecting correctional staff and surrounding communities, with studies linking county-level incarceration rates in jails to a 6.5% increase in community mortality from infectious diseases (Kajeepeta et al., 2021).

Concentration of Incarceration by Race/Ethnicity

Racial and ethnic disparities remain among the most striking features of US incarceration. For example, although Black and Latinx people make up around 30% of the US population, they account for 51% of the jail population (Essex, 2022). A 2021 report from *The Sentencing Project* found that in 12 states, more than half of the prison population was Black and that in 7 states there was a disparity between black and white imprisonment rates of more than 9:1 (Nellis, 2021). Similar disparities were observed in sentencing severity. For example, in California, people of color and individuals with mental illness were found to have sentencing enhancements disproportionately applied to them (Essex, 2022). In 2022, Black Americans had an imprisonment rate of 911 per 100,000, nearly five times that of white Americans (188 per 100,000) (Carson & Klucknow, 2023). American Indian or Alaska Natives also faced disproportionately high rates (801 per 100,000) (Carson & Klucknow, 2023). Hispanic incarceration rates (426 per 100,000) were lower than previous years but remained double the rate for white Americans (Carson & Klucknow, 2023). Interestingly, non-U.S.

citizens make up a substantial portion of the federal prison population, about 15%, with higher proportions in certain states, including Massachusetts (12%) and Nevada (8%) (Carson & Klucknow, 2023).

The percentage of serious offenses differ by race: Black incarcerated individuals are disproportionately incarcerated for public order offenses (46%), particularly weapon violations; Hispanic individuals for drug offenses (61%); American Indian/Alaska Natives for violent offenses (56%); Asians for drug offenses (46%); and White incarcerated individuals for public order offenses unrelated to weapons (48%) (Carson & Klucknow, 2023).

There exists significant racial and economic disparity at each stage of the criminal justice system in the U.S., ranging from encounters with law enforcement and arrests to convictions and sentencing (Pettit & Sykes, 2015). Black Americans report experiencing police brutality at a rate 3.6 times higher than that reported by white Americans, compounding the cycle of trauma, mental health burden, and incarceration risk (Goff et al., 2016; McLeod et al., 2020). Given these circumstances, it is crucial to investigate the association between race and mental health among incarcerated parents.

Concentration of Incarceration by Gender

Incarceration disproportionately affects females, males, and sexual and gender minority (SGM) persons, each with unique health challenges. Females in prison often face higher rates of anxiety, borderline personality features, somatic concerns, and trauma-related symptoms, while incarcerated males are more likely to have borderline features, trauma-related symptoms, and alcohol-related problems (Drapalski et al., 2009). While there were no reported differences in seeking help prior to incarceration, females are more likely to seek and be enrolled in jail-based treatment (Drapalski et al., 2009). On the other hand, SGM persons are at an elevated risk for severe health-related issues from internalized homophobia and discrimination (Baćak et al., 2018).

Until the National Inmate Survey (NIS) became mandated in 2003 by the Prison Rape Elimination Act, jails and prisons did not collect information on sexual orientation, gender identity, and same-sex behaviors (Baćak et al., 2018). From an NIS survey collected in 2011 and 2012, it was estimated that approximately 238,000 SGM persons were incarcerated in the U.S. (Baćak et al., 2018; Meyer et al., 2017). While lesbian, gay, or bisexual (LGB)-identified persons only make up an estimated 2–6% of the general population, they experience incarceration rates over three times higher than the general population (1882 vs. 612 adults per 100,000) (Baćak et al., 2018; Gates, 2011). Transgender persons are also at high risk for victimization in prison, particularly when housed according to birth sex rather than gender identity (Sumner & Jenness, 2014). It was reported that 1 in 3 transgender persons was victimized while incarcerated, with assault rates as high as 59% in male prisons (Beck et al., 2013).

Transgender persons who self-identify as a sexual minority are at even greater risk of victimization and their needs should be further explored (Baćak et al., 2018). In 2012, the Prison Rape Elimination Act required correctional staff to consider the gender identity and personal safety of transgender incarcerated individuals before assigning them to a correctional facility (Baćak et al., 2018). However, these guidelines were not legally binding, and enforcement remains inconsistent (Baćak et al., 2018; US Department of Justice Final Rule. National standards to prevent, 2012). Oftentimes SGM persons conceal their identity or orientation during incarceration to avoid the amplified risks of violence and discrimination in correctional facilities (Baćak et al., 2018). Jails and prisons often enforce traditional sexuality and gender norms, making internalized homo- and transphobia more of a challenging issue during confinement, leading to especially poor health outcomes for current and formerly incarcerated SGM persons (Baćak et al., 2018; Gorga, 2017; Newcomb & Mustanski, 2010).

Concentration of Incarceration by Age

A study found that formerly incarcerated older adults had high levels of depressive symptoms and physical disabilities, with women, especially women of color, facing greater health burdens (Latham-Mintus et al., 2023). As incarcerated populations age, promoting health interventions for different age groups becomes increasingly critical (Latham-Mintus et al., 2023).

In 2022, 19% of incarcerated individuals were under 30, 65% were aged 30–54, and 16% were 55 or older (Carson & Klucknow, 2023). Persons ages 35–39 had the highest imprisonment rate at 832 per 100,000 U.S. residents (Carson & Klucknow, 2023). Moreover, young black males ages 18–19 faced the highest incarceration rates (340 per 100,000), far exceeding rates for other racial groups; this rate is 26 times that of Asian males, 11 times that of white males, 4 times that of Hispanic males, and 2 times that of American Indian or Alaska Native males (Carson & Klucknow, 2023).

In every U.S. state, youth under 18 can be prosecuted and incarcerated as adults, with some states allowing children as young as 12 to be tried as adults (Semenza et al., 2024). Markedly, youth of any age can be imprisoned alongside adults in states like Idaho, Indiana, and Maine (*Interstate Commission for Youth Age Matrix*, 2024; Semenza et al., 2024). Children incarcerated in adult facilities have a much greater risk for early death and have a 33% increase in mortality risk (Semenza et al., 2024; Silver et al., 2023). Compared to children in youth facilities, they also have higher rates of depression, fear, and post-traumatic stress disorder and face a higher risk for physical and sexual assault victimization as well as suicide (Semenza et al., 2024). Many incarcerated youths have unaddressed mental health needs as adult institutions often lack appropriate services to properly treat children (Ng et al., 2012; Semenza et al., 2024). This often has devastating consequences for youth in critical developmental periods, who often face social isolation and experience more severe and more frequent disciplinary action than adults (Kuanliang et al., 2008). Strikingly, 27 states and federal prisons reported holding at least one-person age 17 or younger in their prison facilities in 2022 (Carson & Klucknow, 2023). Addressing age-related disparities is urgent, as incarcerated youth face heightened risk of abuse, physical and mental health challenges, and recidivism. Policies must consider the unique developmental, educational, and safety needs of these young individuals.

Consequences for Communities

As the U.S. leads the world in the number of incarcerated citizens per capita, it is important to examine how incarceration impacts the entirety of the family system (Murphey & Cooper, 2015). Incarceration is concentrated in communities already severely disadvantaged, and its physical and mental impacts extend beyond the incarcerated individual to entire families and communities (Travis, 2014). For example, the incarceration of a family member is linked to family stress, stigma, ambiguous loss, decreased communication, financial strain, feelings of shame, and guilt (Tadros & Presley, 2024) which can lead to various mental health issues, chronic stress and unstable family dynamics (Bruns, 2020). Even before incarceration, families with incarcerated members experience worse outcomes than those without (Lee & Wildeman, 2021).

Children are often the most affected by parental incarceration. More than five million children in the U.S. have or have had a parent incarcerated during their youth (Rhodes et al., 2023). Youth exposed to familial incarceration are more likely to experience multiple stressful life events, including traumatic separation, loneliness, stigma, unstable childcare arrangements, strained parenting, reduced income, and home, school, and neighborhood moves (Murray et al., 2012). These youth are at increased risk for a range of adverse behavioral outcomes (Jackson et al., 2021). Before the age of 14, youth with incarcerated parents are three times as likely to initiate drug and alcohol use and four times as likely to report past-month heroin or prescription pain medication use without a doctor's prescription (Rhodes et al., 2023; Swedo et al., 2020). In the long term, these youth are more likely to engage in risky health behaviors, such as illicit drug and alcohol use, and to experience mental health problems, including depression, as adults (Rhodes et al., 2023).

Some therapies have been found to be helpful in mitigating the stress and negative health impacts of incarceration. For example, mindfulness training, purposefully focusing on the present moment without judgment or the desire for change, has increasingly become popular among both the public and researchers (Pillay & Eagle, 2021). It has been shown to significantly benefit individuals experiencing chronic anxiety, depression, or stress (Pillay & Eagle, 2021). Moreover, Trauma-Focused Cognitive-Behavioral Therapy (TF-CBT) is a trauma-focused therapeutic model that can be integrated into family visits and counseling sessions as a coping strategy to help children with depression, anger, aggression, isolating behaviors, and self-harming behaviors (Cohen & Mannarino, 2015; Malik et al., 2023; Morgan-Mullane, 2018). Finally, as incarcerated individuals age, sustained programs focused on recidivism prevention, healthcare continuity, housing, access to health insurance, disability, increased funding, and social support are critical to ensure that resources are available for successful reentry into communities (Onyeali et al., 2023).

Why You Should Care About Mass Incarceration

Countless studies have shown that incarceration can lead to lower family functioning, impaired social networks, decreased graduation rates, decreased employment rates, increased violence and victimization, physical and mental health consequences, and a significant decrease in relational satisfaction. Unfortunately, criminal justice settings often lack mental health professionals trained in family and couples therapy, limiting access to crucial psychoeducation and relational support. Mental health professionals can help families learn and develop tools to create stable and supportive environments by teaching healthy communication skills, conflict resolution, empathy, and systematic reframing of problems.

Presently, the coronavirus pandemic has caused mental health professionals to provide more telehealth services (Zangani et al., 2022). However, there was still the challenge of determining how to deliver relationship-oriented services to underserved populations that are often forgotten during crises, including incarcerated individuals and their families. The pandemic has seemingly ended, but the need for relational mental health care in corrections, where families are separated and not able to see each other, will continue. We must advocate for incarcerated individuals and their families to have access to these services. However, much more work needs to be done to allow for telehealth to be the norm versus an emergency alternative. The hope is that what began as a response to the pandemic can also contribute to the normalization and destigmatization of engaging in mental health services in corrections.

Racial and ethnic disparities in incarceration reflect systemic injustices tied to lack of resources, poverty, stigma, and weaker family dynamics. We advocate adopting an *incarcerated informed lens, a term we coined to* acknowledge both unintended and intended consequences of incarceration (racial disparities, employment, education, poverty, health, and relationships) (Tadros et al., 2021). Policy makers should also address the policing and justice policies that serve to incarcerate more people of color. This racial disparity deserves attention, and the future of these individuals calls for more equalized opportunities for success. Future challenges for researchers and policy makers will be to examine the best methods to support individuals prior to incarceration instead of waiting and relying on visitation and correctional services. This starts with understanding systemic problems such as racism, poverty, and mass incarceration from a historical and multi-institutional context. We need to consider the broader perspective; reducing mass incarceration can help in improving mental, physical, and relational health, reducing recidivism, and lessening the stigma. Stronger families equal stronger communities.

References

Annette Gordon-Reed. *Illinois State Commission on Criminal Justice and Sentencing Reform.* (2016).

Annette Gordon-Reed. *Interstate Commission for Youth Age Matrix.* (2024). https://juvenilecompact.org/age-matrix

Baćak, V., Thurman, K., Eyer, K., Qureshi, R., Bird, J. D. P., Rivera, L. M., & Kim, S. A. (2018). Incarceration as a health determinant for sexual orientation and gender minority persons. *American Journal of Public Health, 108*(8), 994–999. https://doi.org/10.2105/ajph.2018.304500

Beck, A. J., Berzofsky, M., Caspar, R., & Krebs, C. (2013). Sexual victimization in prisons and jails reported by inmates, 2011–12. *NCJ*, 241399.

Bruns, A. (2020). Partner incarceration and financial support from kin. *Journal of Family Issues, 41*(11), 2112–2135.

Carson, E. A., & Klucknow, R. (2023). *Prisoners in 2022 – Statistical tables.* https://bjs.ojp.gov/media/document/70441

Cloud, D. H., Drucker, E., Browne, A., & Parsons, J. (2015). Public health and solitary confinement in the United States. *American Journal of Public Health, 105*(1), 18–26. https://doi.org/10.2105/AJPH.2014.302205

Cohen, J. A., & Mannarino, A. P. (2015). Trauma-focused cognitive behavioral therapy for traumatized children and families. *Child and Adolescent Psychiatric Clinics of North America, 24*(3), 557.

Collier, L. (2014, October 1). Incarceration nation. *Monitor on Psychology, 45*(9). https://www.apa.org/monitor/2014/10/incarceration

Drapalski, A. L., Youman, K., Stuewig, J., & Tangney, J. (2009). Gender differences in jail inmates' symptoms of mental illness, treatment history and treatment seeking. *Criminal Behaviour and Mental Health, 19*(3), 193–206. https://doi.org/10.1002/cbm.733

Essex, A. H. (2022). *Justice racial and ethnic disparities in the justice system* (The Legislative Primer Series for Front-End, Issue. https://www.ncsl.org/civil-and-criminal-justice/racial-and-ethnic-disparities-in-the-criminal-justice-system

Fazel, S., Hayes, A. J., Bartellas, K., Clerici, M., & Trestman, R. (2016). Mental health of prisoners: Prevalence, adverse outcomes, and interventions. *The Lancet Psychiatry*, *3*(9), 871–881. https://doi.org/10.1016/S2215-0366(16)30142-0

Gates, G. (2011). *How many people are lesbian, gay, bisexual, and transgender?* https://williamsinstitute.law.ucla.edu/publications/adult-lgbt-pop-us/

Goff, P. A., Lloyd, T., Geller, A., Raphael, S., & Glaser, J. (2016). *The science of justice: Race, arrests and police use of force*. Center for Policing Equity. Available: https://policingequity.org/images/pdfs-doc/CPE_SoJ_Race-Arrests-UoF_2016-07-08-1130.pdf

Gorga, A. (2017). "Kinda like a man and a woman thing": The construction and reification of gender hegemony in a women's prison. *Social Currents*, *4*(5), 413–428.

Gur-Arie, M. (2022). *Incarceration*. Judiciaries Worldwide. https://judiciaries-worldwide.fjc.gov/incarceration#:~:text=According%20to%20the%20World%20Population%20Review%2C%20as,Indonesia%20(266%2C259)%2C%20Mexico%20(220%2C866)%2C%20and%20Iran%20(189%2C000).

Harrison, A. J., Jakubowski, J. A., Abram, K. M., Teplin, L. A., & Welty, L. J. (2020). Patterns of incarceration among youth after detention: A 16-year longitudinal study. *Children and Youth Services Review*, *108*, 104516. https://doi.org/https://doi.org/10.1016/j.childyouth.2019.104516

Jackson, D. B., Testa, A., Semenza, D. C., & Vaughn, M. G. (2021). Parental incarceration, child adversity, and child health: A strategic comparison approach. *International Journal of Environmental Research and Public Health*, *18*(7), 3384.

Kajeepeta, S., Mauro, P. M., Keyes, K. M., El-Sayed, A. M., Rutherford, C. G., & Prins, S. J. (2021). Association between county jail incarceration and cause-specific county mortality in the USA, 1987–2017: A retrospective, longitudinal study. *The Lancet Public Health*, *6*(4), e240–e248. https://doi.org/10.1016/S2468-2667(20)30283-8

Kuanliang, A., Sorensen, J. R., & Cunningham, M. D. (2008). Juvenile inmates in an adult prison system: Rates of disciplinary misconduct and violence. *Criminal Justice and Behavior*, *35*(9), 1186–1201.

Latham-Mintus, K., Deck, M. M., & Nelson, E. (2023). Aging with incarceration histories: An intersectional examination of incarceration and health outcomes among older adults. *The Journals of Gerontology: Series B*, *78*(5), 853–865. https://doi.org/10.1093/geronb/gbac088

Lee, H., & Wildeman, C. (2021). Assessing mass incarceration's effects on families. *Science*, *374*(6565), 277–281. https://doi.org/10.1126/science.abj7777

Leibowitz, A. I., Siedner, M. J., Tsai, A. C., & Mohareb, A. M. (2021). Association between prison crowding and cOVID-19 incidence rates in Massachusetts Prisons, April 2020-January 2021. *JAMA Internal Medicine*, *181*(10), 1315–1321. https://doi.org/10.1001/jamainternmed.2021.4392

Malik, N., Facer-Irwin, E., Dickson, H., Bird, A., & MacManus, D. (2023). The effectiveness of trauma-focused interventions in prison settings: A systematic review and meta-analysis. *Trauma Violence Abuse*, *24*(2), 844–857. https://doi.org/10.1177/15248380211043890

McLeod, M. N., Heller, D., Manze, M. G., & Echeverria, S. E. (2020). Police interactions and the mental health of Black Americans: A systematic review. *Journal of Racial and Ethnic Health Disparities*, *7*, 10–27.

Meyer, I. H., Flores, A. R., Stemple, L., Romero, A. P., Wilson, B. D., & Herman, J. L. (2017). Incarceration rates and traits of sexual minorities in the United States: National inmate survey, 2011–2012. *American Journal of Public Health, 107*(2), 267–273. https://doi.org/10.2105/ajph.2016.303576

Mooney, A. C., Neilands, T. B., Giannella, E., Morris, M. D., Tulsky, J., & Glymour, M. M. (2019). Effects of a voter initiative on disparities in punishment severity for drug offenses across California counties. *Social Science & Medicine, 230*, 9–19. https://doi.org/10.1016/j.socscimed.2019.04.025

Morgan-Mullane, A. (2018). Trauma focused cognitive behavioral therapy with children of incarcerated parents. *Clinical Social Work Journal, 46*(3), 200–209. https://doi.org/10.1007/s10615-017-0642-5

Murphey, D., & Cooper, P. M. (2015). Parents behind bars: What happens to their children? *Child Trends*. https://doi.org/10.13140/RG.2.1.2444.4243

Murray, J., Farrington, D. P., & Sekol, I. (2012). Children's antisocial behavior, mental health, drug use, and educational performance after parental incarceration: A systematic review and meta-analysis. *Psychol Bull, 138*(2), 175–210. https://doi.org/10.1037/a0026407

Nellis, A. (2021). *The color of justice: Racial and ethnic disparity in state prisons*. The Sentencing Project. https://www.sentencingproject.org/reports/the-color-of-justice-racial-and-ethnic-disparity-in-state-prisons-the-sentencing-project/

Newcomb, M. E., & Mustanski, B. (2010). Internalized homophobia and internalizing mental health problems: A meta-analytic review. *Clinical Psychology Review, 30*(8), 1019–1029.

Ng, I. Y., Sarri, R. C., Shook, J. J., & Stoffregen, E. (2012). Comparison of correctional services for youth incarcerated in adult and juvenile facilities in Michigan. *The Prison Journal, 92*(4), 460–483.

Onyeali, R., Howell, B. A., McInnes, D. K., Emerson, A., & Williams, M. E. (2023). The case for transitional services and programs for older adults reentering society: A narrative review of US departments of correction and recommendations. *International Journal of Prisoner Health, 19*(1), 4–19. https://doi.org/10.1108/ijph-08-2021-0073

Pettit, B., & Sykes, B. L. (2015). Civil rights legislation and legalized exclusion: Mass incarceration and the masking of inequality. *Sociological Forum, 30*(S1), 589–611. https://doi.org/10.1111/socf.12179

Pillay, K., & Eagle, G. (2021). The case for mindfulness interventions for traumatic stress in high violence, low resource settings. *Current Psychology: A Journal for Diverse Perspectives on Diverse Psychological Issues, 40*(5), 2400–2414. https://doi.org/10.1007/s12144-019-00177-1

Reiter, K., Ventura, J., Lovell, D., Augustine, D., Barragan, M., Blair, T., Chesnut, K., Dashtgard, P., Gonzalez, G., Pifer, N., & Strong, J. (2020). Psychological distress in solitary confinement: Symptoms, severity, and prevalence in the United States, 2017–2018. *American Journal of Public Health, 110*(S56-S62). https://doi.org/10.2105/AJPH.2019.305375

Rhodes, C. A., Thomas, N., O'Hara, K. L., Hita, L., Blake, A., Wolchik, S. A., Fisher, B., Freeman, M., Chen, D., & Berkel, C. (2023). Enhancing the focus: How does parental incarceration fit into the overall picture of Adverse Childhood Experiences

(ACEs) and Positive Childhood Experiences (PCEs)? *Research on Child and Adolescent Psychopathology*, *51*(12), 1933–1944. https://doi.org/10.1007/s10802-023-01142-0

Semenza, D. C., Silver, I. A., & Jackson, D. B. (2024). Youth incarceration in adult facilities and mental health in early adulthood. *Journal of Adolescent Health*, *74*(5), 989–995. https://doi.org/10.1016/j.jadohealth.2024.01.008

Shannon, S. K., Uggen, C., Schnittker, J., Thompson, M., Wakefield, S., & Massoglia, M. (2017). The growth, scope, and spatial distribution of people with felony records in the United States, 1948–2010. *Demography*, *54*(5), 1795–1818. https://doi.org/10.1007/s13524-017-0611-1

Silver, I. A., Semenza, D. C., & Nedelec, J. L. (2023). Incarceration of youths in an adult correctional facility and risk of premature death. *JAMA Network Open*, *6*(7), e2321805–e2321805.

Substance Abuse Treatment: For Adults in the Criminal Justice System: 9 Treatment Issues Specific to Prisons. (2005). https://www.ncbi.nlm.nih.gov/books/NBK572935/

Sumner, J., & Jenness, V. (2014). Gender integration in sex-segregated prisons. In D. Peterson & V. R. Panfil (Eds.), *Handbook of LGBT communities, crime, and justice* (pp. 229–260). Springer.

Swavola, E. R. K., & Subramanian, R. (2016). *Overlooked: Women and jails in an era of reform.* Vera Institute of Justice. https://www.vera.org/publications/overlooked-women-and-jails-report

Swedo, E. A., Sumner, S. A., de Fijter, S., Werhan, L., Norris, K., Beauregard, J. L., Montgomery, M. P., Rose, E. B., Hillis, S. D., & Massetti, G. M. (2020). Adolescent opioid misuse attributable to adverse childhood experiences. *The Journal of Pediatrics*, *224*, 102–109. e103.

Tadros, E., Hutcherson, R., & Greene, A. (2021). Advocating for an incarcerated informed lens in therapy. *International Journal of Offender Therapy and Comparative Criminology*, *65*(5), 631–643. https://doi.org/10.1177/0306624X20975162

Tadros, E., & Presley, S. (2024). "Fear of the Unknown": Coparenting with an incarcerated individual. *International Journal of Offender Therapy & Comparative Criminology*, *68*(6–7) 693–712. https://doi.org/10.1177/0306624X221106335

Travis, J. W. B., & Redburn, S. (2014). *The growth of incarceration in the United States: Exploring causes and consequences.* National Academies Press.

US Department of Justice Final Rule. National standards to prevent, d., and respond to prison rape under the Prison Rape Elimination Act (PREA). 2012. (2012). https://www.prearesourcecenter.org/sites/default/files/content/prisonsandjailsfinalstandards_0.pd.

Zangani, C., Ostinelli, E. G., Smith, K. A., Hong, J. S. W., Macdonald, O., Reen, G., Reid, K., Vincent, C., Syed Sheriff, R., Harrison, P. J., Hawton, K., Pitman, A., Bale, R., Fazel, S., Geddes, J. R., & Cipriani, A. (2022). Impact of the COVID-19 pandemic on the global delivery of mental health services and telemental health: Systematic review. *JMIR Mental Health*, *9*(8), e38600. https://doi.org/10.2196/38600

Chapter 2

Race, Ethnicity, Incarceration, and the Family in the United States

Katherine A. Durante and Hibba Ahmed

Nearly 50 years ago, the United States began an unprecedented era of mass incarceration – a term commonly used to describe the extreme U.S. imprisonment rates relative to other nations and historical standards, making it the world leader in prison and jail population sizes and per capita. In 1980, there were fewer than 330,000 people incarcerated in U.S. state and federal prisons (Vera Institute of Justice, 2024). Rapid annual growth led to a peak prison population of more than 1.6 million people in 2009, followed by a slow decline over the next decade, which accelerated during the 2020 COVID-19 pandemic. Approximately 660 per 100,000 adult U.S. residents were incarcerated in prisons or jails in 2020, marking a substantial reduction compared to 960 per 100,000 only a decade earlier (Kluckow & Zeng, 2022). However, the most recent U.S. prison and jail population numbers indicate a return to growth in 2022 (Vera Institute of Justice,≈2024).

Mass incarceration removes millions of people from their families and communities while, in turn, harming their mental and physical health (e.g., Kouyoumdjian et al., 2016) and prospects of employment and earnings (e.g., Gordon et al., 2023), among other detrimental consequences. Likewise, the consequences for left-behind partners can be monumental, causing worsened health and well-being (Wildeman et al., 2012, 2013), financial and housing insecurity (Geller & Franklin, 2014; Harman et al., 2007), and isolation (Harman et al., 2007). Left-behind children face academic risks (McLeod et al., 2019) and exhibit problem behavior (Geller et al., 2009). Thus, the adverse consequences associated with incarceration extend well beyond individuals, affecting families, communities, and society at large. Black, low-income, and other marginalized communities have been particularly devastated by mass incarceration. In this chapter, we outline trends, disparities, and causes of imprisonment, followed by their implications for individuals, families, and communities. We then discuss future directions.

DOI: 10.4324/9781003542940-2

Incarceration Trends: Race, Ethnicity, Gender, and Social Class

The social costs of incarceration are distributed unequally across U.S. society. Black American adults were incarcerated in prisons at a rate of 901 per 100,000 in 2021, compared to 181 per 100,000 White American adults and 72 per 100,000 Asian American adults (Prison Policy Initiative, 2024). American Indian/Alaskan Native (AI/AN) and Latino adults fell in between with an estimated 763 and 434 per 100,000 persons incarcerated, respectively. Nearly 1 in 5 Black men born in 2001 will be imprisoned at some point in their lives, a substantial decline from the 1981 Black male birth cohort, who experienced a 1 in 3 lifetime risk of incarceration (Robey et al., 2023). The imprisonment rate for Black men declined by 44% between 1999 and 2019, reducing the still-high imprisonment racial disparity to about 6-to-1 Black men to White men (Robey et al., 2023).

The mass incarceration era has also led to a historically high number of women in jails and prisons. Women make up less than 10% of incarcerated people in the United States, yet their increased presence in jails and prisons between 1970 and 2015 was even more pronounced than for men. The number of women in prison grew from under 6,000 to approximately 105,000 – a more than 17-fold increase (Nellis, 2024). Black and Latina women are incarcerated at about 1.6 and 1.2 times the rate of White women, respectively (Budd, 2024). AI/AN women comprise 2.5% of the female prison and local jail populations, despite only making up 0.7% of the U.S. female population (Prison Policy Initiative, 2024).

Social class is also related to incarceration; the prison population primarily draws from the lowest socioeconomic groups in society (Western & Pettit, 2010). Young Black men with limited education and who derive from disadvantaged urban communities are vastly overrepresented in U.S. jails and prisons, leading some to argue that "hyperincarceration" more accurately characterizes the past 50 years of imprisonment trends (e.g., Wacquant, 2010). The neighborhoods that these men come from are incarceration "hot spots" (Sampson & Loeffler, 2010, p. 20) and often have high levels of poverty, unemployment, family disruption, and racial isolation. They have higher incarceration rates even when controlling for crime, which suggests that systemic disadvantage keeps residents trapped in a negative self-reinforcing cycle (Sampson & Loeffler, 2010). Race, class, residential location, and incarceration are inextricably linked, and the most vulnerable and disadvantaged persons are particularly susceptible to the policies that have driven mass incarceration.

The Rise of Mass Incarceration and Racial/Ethnic Disparities

A piecemeal approach to policy has driven the massive prison population growth. State and federal legislators in the 1980s and 1990s passed laws aimed at increasing the likelihood of a prison sentence following a criminal conviction and requiring individuals to spend more time behind bars, especially for violent and drug convictions (Redburn et al., 2014). Approximately 87% of individuals incarcerated in U.S. prisons are housed in state facilities, while only about 13% are under the jurisdiction of the federal government (Carson & Kluckow, 2023). The federal government has limited direct impact on mass incarceration; however, it serves as a model for states to follow and has influenced "tough on crime" laws nationally (Ofer, 2019). For example, the 1984 Sentencing Reform Act established long mandatory minimum sentences for many federal crimes and served as a template that states followed (Cullen, 2018). Such laws remove or limit judicial discretion and require defendants convicted of certain crimes to serve at least the minimum prison time mandated by law.

Another driver of mass incarceration is the Violent Crime Control and Law Enforcement Act of 1994, more commonly known as the 1994 Crime Bill. It incentivized states to pass increasingly punitive measures, such as habitual offender and truth-in-sentencing laws, and to build more prisons (Ofer, 2019). "Three-strikes" laws remove judicial discretion and require repeat offenders to receive a severe penalty, such as life imprisonment, after being convicted of three crimes. Habitual offender laws have led to severe, disproportionate punishment for people convicted of relatively minor offenses that would not normally merit such a harsh sentence (Cullen, 2018). The federal government offered prison expansion grants to states to pass truth-in-sentencing laws, which require individuals to serve at least 85% of their prison sentence before becoming eligible for parole. Such laws have led to larger prison populations by requiring more time spent in prison regardless of good behavior or rehabilitation (Bureau of Justice Administration, 2022).

Rising violent crime rates, paired with public support for punitive policies, also encouraged a concurrent shift in prosecutorial decision-making (Pfaff, 2017). Unlike judges, prosecutors have few limits on their discretion. Moreover, district attorneys are elected officials with an incentive to act tough on crime and appease their constituents. Starting in the mid-1990s, prosecutors doubled the rate of felony charges brought against defendants, using their immense power to increase incarceration even as crime rates declined (Pfaff, 2017).

There is little dispute that crime control policies and practices have driven incarceration rates, but there is less consensus on why they took hold (Beckett & Francis, 2020). The impact on crime reduction and deterrence has diminishing returns as imprisonment rates rise (Liedka et al., 2006). Moreover, exposure to the prison environment is considered criminogenic, potentially increasing crime (Vieraitis et al., 2007). The punitive policy shift occurred following the successes achieved by the civil rights movement. Scholars contend that electoral politics, a backlash to racial gains, and other social dynamics, such as inequality, the rise of neoliberalism and market deregulation, and the increase in violent crime, facilitated these policies (Beckett & Francis, 2020; Garland, 2001; Hagan, 2010; Hinton, 2020; Wacquant, 2010). For example, Wacquant (2010) argues that the United States shifted social spending to build a large penal state, while cutting the social welfare state and criminalizing poverty, in turn creating a large underclass of insecure labor, primarily lower-class Black men from disadvantaged urban areas. Garland (2001) argues that changes in cultural values underlie the choice to mass incarcerate, including a declining interest in rehabilitation, increased support for retribution, the dehumanization of those who commit crime, and the emergence of fear of crime, support for victims, and demands for feeling safe and secure. Others emphasize the role of racial resentment, such as the successful cultural conflation of Black Americans as inherently dangerous and criminal (Beckett & Francis, 2020; Hinton, 2020).

Causes of Disparity

Racial and ethnic incarceration disparities are well-documented in all 50 states and the federal prison system. The drivers of these disparities are complex, with several contributing factors, primarily rooted in the social inequality that has characterized U.S. society both past and present. The contemporary penal system can be traced back to slavery, with several legal mechanisms enacted to maintain White racial supremacy (Alexander, 2010). Differences in criminal offending, which reflect both the behaviors lawmakers have criminalized and the outcomes of structural inequalities, are also key drivers of disparity. Empirical research also suggests that biases in the criminal justice system contact and processing can lead to unfavorable sentencing outcomes, especially for young Black men.

Scholars argue that racial disparity in the contemporary U.S. criminal legal system is rooted in a historically evolving legal framework that promotes racial inequality and the systemic oppression of Black Americans (Alexander, 2010). The 13th Amendment (1865) abolished slavery and involuntary servitude with one exception – punishment for crime. Convict leasing and prison farms followed, along with Black Codes, which criminalized the behavior of Black Americans through vagrancy laws, leading to their arrest and exploitation (Alexander, 2010). Jim Crow laws after Reconstruction maintained racial hierarchy through mandated segregation in the South until the U.S. Supreme Court overturned their legality in the historic *Brown v. Board of Education* (1954) ruling. Still, racialized control continued as racial stereotypes and fear of crime fueled harsher policing, particularly following the Great Migration of the 1970s (Alexander, 2010).

"Law and order" rhetoric aimed at civil rights activism informed many of the policies that expanded the prison population, particularly for minoritized men. The war on drugs has led to excessive disparities in arrest and incarceration. For example, the notorious 100-to-1 crack v. powder cocaine sentencing disparity that triggered a mandatory minimum sentence (later reduced to 18-to-1 by the Fair Sentencing Act of 2010) established under the 1986 Anti-Drug Abuse Act led to disproportionate incarceration and lengthy prison sentences for Black Americans (The United States Sentencing Commission, 2007). Drug offenders make up only a minority of state prison populations. Yet, punitive drug laws have led Alexander (2010) and others to argue that the drug war has created an underclass or "caste" system akin to Jim Crow law, with Black Americans becoming disproportionately branded as drug felons. The felony label subsequently restricts their access to employment, housing, political participation, and other opportunities.

Moreover, racial segregation persists in many U.S. cities. White Americans generally live in neighborhoods with an abundance of resources and opportunities. Black Americans, and to a lesser extent Latinos, often live in disadvantaged communities characterized by high levels of crime, residential turnover, and police surveillance, along with a lack of investment in housing and infrastructure, access to good jobs and schools, and other criminogenic characteristics (Massey, 2016). Thus, the different neighborhood conditions in which Americans live are crucial drivers of differences in criminal offending, especially regarding violent crime (Krivo et al., 2021). For example, in 2010, White neighborhoods had about 1.4 violent crimes per 1,000 residents compared to 2.9 per 1,000 residents in Latino and multiethnic neighborhoods and 8.5 per 1,000 residents in Black neighborhoods (Krivo et al., 2021). Neighborhood segregation has allowed concentrated disadvantage to flourish in predominantly non-White neighborhoods, which in turn drives racial and ethnic disparities in crime rates, incarceration, exposure to neighborhood and community violence, and social disorder, operating as a feedback loop (Krivo et al., 2021; Sampson & Loeffler, 2010).

Disparity also arises from the many decisions made between initial police contact and sentencing. "Accumulated disadvantage" describes the sequence where earlier adverse events or decisions in criminal legal case processing increase the odds of later adverse events or decisions occurring (Wooldredge et al., 2015). For example, longer pretrial detention can increase the odds of conviction (Martinez et al., 2020). Unsurprisingly, young Black and Latino men are the most vulnerable as they may be viewed as particularly dangerous or blameworthy by prosecutors or judges (Martinez et al., 2020; Wooldredge et al., 2015). These stereotypes may especially disadvantage young men of color during sentencing (Freiburger et al., 2019). Several studies find that Black and Latino defendants receive slightly to moderately longer sentences than their White counterparts (e.g., Durante, 2021; Steffensmeier et al., 2017), although the findings of Latino/White disparity are less consistent (e.g., Jordan & Freiburger, 2015).

Collateral Consequences of Incarceration

The prison experience can lead to enduring and often devastating consequences for individuals during community reentry and long after. The separation from society, the poor and overcrowded living conditions, and exposure to violence can be damaging to mental health. For example, posttraumatic stress disorder (PTSD) can arise from abuse, solitary confinement, and coercion during imprisonment (Piper & Berle, 2019). Anxiety, mood, impulse control, and substance abuse disorders are each prevalent among formerly incarcerated persons (Schnittker et al., 2012). Incarceration can increase the post-release odds of depression and mental health concerns (Porter & DeMarco, 2018). Some evidence points to a unique post-incarceration syndrome that includes symptoms of PTSD, institutionalized personality traits, social–sensory disorientation, and alienation (Liem & Kunst, 2013). Still, mental health challenges, criminal offending, and the likelihood of incarceration are each strongly related to childhood experiences, and the criminalization of mental health disorders can lead to imprisonment.

Incarceration may temporarily improve physical health by providing essential services, such as health care, housing, and food, to vulnerable populations (National Research Council and Institute of Medicine, 2013). Prisons might also protect young Black men from excess mortality caused by external factors such as homicides and accidents (Rosen et al., 2011). Still, incarceration is associated with poor or worsened post-release health. Formerly incarcerated individuals experience excess premature mortality (Kouyoumdjian et al., 2016) and suicide (Pratt et al., 2006) and have higher prevalences of physical limitations (Latham-Mintus et al, 2023) and illness than the general population, such as infectious diseases (Massoglia, 2008), hypertension (Wang et al., 2009), and obesity (Houle, 2014).

Separation from society can lead to psychological detachment and social isolation from family and friends (Harman et al., 2007). Incarcerated and previously incarcerated individuals experience a reduced chance of marriage (Huebner, 2005) and a heightened risk of relationship dissolution, including divorce (Apel et al., 2010; Siennick et al., 2013). Restrictions on autonomy and decision-making while in prison can harm the parent-child relationship (Swanson et al., 2013; Tasca, 2016).

Economic hardship is common during community reentry and onward. The unemployment rate of this group is estimated to be about five times higher than that of the general population (Couloute & Kopf, 2018). Black men with criminal records are particularly likely to face employment discrimination, compounding the employment discrimination that they already experience (Pager et al., 2009). Sustained detachment from the labor force and opportunities to earn more income through illicit means may discourage individuals from seeking legitimate employment (Apel & Sweeten,

2010). Moreover, incarcerated men from neighborhoods with poor economic opportunities have worse perceptions of post-release employability (Roddy & Durante, 2024), which may be discouraging. Wages are suppressed for those who find paid labor; incarceration may lead to a 50% reduction in lifetime earnings (Gordon et al., 2023).

Access to safe and affordable housing is hindered by both structural and individual barriers, which result from and are exacerbated by economic hardship. For example, public housing bans for individuals with felonies, discrimination in the private rental market, and parole requirements that include stringent housing criteria restrict options (Augustine & Kushel, 2022). Co-occurring problems like mental illness, substance abuse, and fragile family relationships can also drive housing insecurity (Herbert et al., 2015).

Incarceration can also lead to a reduction in civic and political participation. Being incarcerated or having a felony conviction triggers voting restrictions or bans on individuals in 48 states (Uggen et al., 2024). For example, in 2024, more than 4 million Americans, or 1.7% of the voting population, were ineligible to vote because of their criminal history. Black Americans are disproportionately disenfranchised, especially in Florida, Arizona, Kentucky, South Dakota, and Tennessee (Uggen et al., 2024). These restrictions suppress political participation and representation among those who are among the most underrepresented and underserved, limiting their opportunities for self-advocacy.

Consequences for Families

Incarceration is also associated with detrimental outcomes for the partners and children of people in prison. The separation can cause emotional withdrawal, relationship instability, a decline in relationship quality, isolation, or stigma (DeHart et al., 2018; Harman et al., 2007; Turney, 2015). The high financial costs for visitation and phone calls can lead to strain in relationships (Durante et al., 2024). These extra costs occur at a time when budgets are already tight, as the removal of a partner or parent from the home can cause financial hardship for family members (Arditti et al., 2003; DeHart et al., 2018; Harman et al., 2007).

The subsequent reduction in family income can lead to housing and food insecurity (Geller & Franklin, 2014; Testa & Jackson, 2020), a loss of child support and other social supports (Arditti et al., 2003; Harman et al., 2007), and force partners – who are usually women – to pick up additional employment, extra hours, or sell belongings to pay bills (Bruns, 2019; DeHart et al., 2018). The resulting stress can be damaging to mental and physical health. Depressive symptoms and suboptimal mental health are common among individuals with incarcerated partners or other family members (Tadros, Durante, Morgan, et al., 2022; Turney, 2021; Wildeman et al., 2012). Hazardous alcohol consumption and substance abuse may arise (Wildeman et al., 2013). Nonincarcerated partners are at an elevated risk of experiencing cardiovascular issues, relative to the general population (Lee et al., 2014; Wildeman et al., 2013). Women with incarcerated family members have an increased risk of obesity, heart attacks, and strokes (Lee et al., 2014). Nonincarcerated women may experience worse health than their incarcerated partners (Tadros, Durante, McKay, et al., 2022). The spread of sexually transmitted infections (STIs), the human immunodeficiency virus (HIV), and acquired immune deficiency syndrome (AIDS) is a concern during reentry due to higher prevalences within prisons and risky sexual behavior (Comfort et al., 2005; Harman et al., 2007).

Children who experience family incarceration are nearly three times more likely than their peers to engage in risky health behaviors and have more than twice the odds of being diagnosed with a mental health or behavioral problem (Provencher & Conway, 2019). Adults who experienced family incarceration as a child are about 50% more likely to experience physical health problems compared to their peers. Childhood stress caused by parental incarceration can harm health and well-being across the life course. Children with incarcerated parents are also more likely to exhibit poor academic performance, such as lower vocabulary development (McLeod et al., 2019) and grade retention (Horton, 2022), and the stigma from parental incarceration can drive isolation from peers (Saunders, 2018). Parental incarceration can cause behavioral problems, early juvenile delinquency, and juvenile justice involvement, particularly among boys (Geller et al., 2009, 2012; Horton, 2022; Provencher & Conway, 2019; Turney, 2017). These adverse outcomes are disproportionately felt by Black and Latino youth since they are more likely to experience familial incarceration. In 2021, Black and Latino youth were 4.7 and 2.1 times more likely to be placed in juvenile facilities compared to White youth, respectively (Rovner, 2023a, 2023b). This disparity reinforces the cycle in which parental incarceration can increase the risk of youth incarceration, maintaining intergenerational disadvantage.

Finally, incarceration can also provide an opportunity for positive changes for families. Time spent in prison can facilitate reflection on relationships (Turney, 2015) and help couples improve their communication (DeHart et al., 2018) and romance (Comfort, 2008). Moreover, it provides an avenue to work on relationship problems in a safe environment in situations where the incarcerated person is physically or financially abusive and might be the only opportunity for self-improvement services like substance abuse or family violence classes (Comfort, 2008).

Consequences for Communities

Racial and ethnic disparities in incarceration – although themselves largely a product of inequality in society – drive other inequalities across communities, such as income, wealth, and population health disparities. Black families, for example, are disproportionately hurt by the high costs of having a loved one incarcerated, including the loss of a wage earner, expensive fines and fees owed to courts and other criminal justice system entities, and relationship maintenance expenses. These challenges persist beyond release from prison, as lifelong barriers to employment and earnings contribute to the overall Black-White income and wealth gaps (Gordon et al., 2023). Moreover, formerly incarcerated people often reenter and reside in the same neighborhoods (Clear, 2008), which are criminogenic with high levels of unemployment, poverty, and other poor outcomes that drive crime and incarceration (Sampson & Loeffler, 2010). Neighborhood-level studies of population health find that the people and families in these neighborhoods also have higher prevalences of HIV/AIDS, asthma, preterm births, community violence, depression, and other mental health issues (e.g., Jahn et al., 2020; Rogers et al., 2012). Perhaps most alarmingly, experiencing the incarceration of a family member is associated with a 2.6-year reduction in life expectancy, and this reduction may even be bigger among Black Americans (Sundaresh et al., 2021). Any focus on ameliorating racial and ethnic inequality in other domains of society must consider incarceration as a potential contributor and driver of disparity.

Looking Forward

The policies, structural conditions, and historical events that have driven mass incarceration and racial disparities in imprisonment have devastated individuals, families, and communities. Still, there is an opportunity for positive change at the local and policy levels, and in some cases, this work is already happening. Prison programming focused on relationship education, including family functioning, communication, commitment and forgiveness, problem-solving, and similar topics, is a promising pathway for marriage and family therapists, social workers, and clinicians to help strengthen relationships and build resilience (Durante et al., 2023; Harcourt et al., 2017). However, prison programming is often limited to vocational and educational training. The adoption of relationship education programming in prisons presents an untapped resource that can facilitate the success of couples and families in functioning and reintegration (Harcourt et al., 2017). There are also opportunities to expand education and interventions associated with specialized needs for children, family violence, substance abuse, and disease transmission among incarcerated individuals and their family members.

Policy changes at the state and federal levels aimed at decarceration and reducing racial and ethnic disparities in imprisonment have started to address the punitive consequences of laws from the 1980s and 1990s. For example, the Fair Sentencing Act of 2010 reduced the crack-to-powder sentencing disparity to 18-to-1. Some states have made it easier to petition courts for resentencing to reduce prison time (Ghandnoosh et al., 2023). Others have reduced prison admissions by downgrading drug possession charges, and have ended cash bail and other policies that target people with limited financial resources. For example, California's Proposition 47 (2014) and Oklahoma's State Question 780 (2016) each reclassified select low-level, nonviolent offenses from felonies to misdemeanors. Other promising policies include curbing truth-in-sentencing laws, reducing sentencing enhancements, and moving away from mandatory minimums (Ghandnoosh et al., 2023).

Recreational cannabis is now legal in 24 states and Washington, D.C., as of 2024. The early research on these policies suggests that cannabis arrests have plummeted in these jurisdictions, although racial disparities in arrests and subsequent jail and prison incarcerations persist (Firth et al., 2019; Wu et al., 2023, 2024). These findings demonstrate the importance of lawmakers being purposeful when writing legislation targeted at reducing disparity. For example, in addition to decriminalizing or legalizing cannabis, adopting laws that expunge previous criminal convictions for cannabis is a necessary step for racial justice since criminal history is a key determinant of sentencing. Purposeful efforts to divert more people of color to drug treatment programs instead of prison can also reduce disparity while potentially reducing future offending and improving public health (Nicosia, 2013).

Conclusion

This chapter provided an overview of incarceration trends in the United States, emphasizing its relationship with race, ethnicity, and the family unit. Despite decades of social progress and recent positive criminal justice reforms, mass incarceration, racial disparity, and damaging consequences to individuals, families, and communities persist. Policies and practices at the local level – such as correctional facilities adopting or expanding relationship education programming or counties expanding specialty court diversion programming – and at the state and national levels – such as proactive laws adopted to reduce jail and prison admissions – provide a variety of potential tools for addressing mass incarceration, racial and ethnic disparity, and the associated collateral consequences.

References

Alexander, M. (2010). *The New Jim Crow: Mass incarceration in the age of colorblindness.* The New Press.

Apel, R., Blokland, A. A. J., Nieuwbeerta, P., & van Schellen, M. (2010). The impact of imprisonment on marriage and divorce: A risk set matching approach. *Journal of Quantitative Criminology, 26*, 269–300. https://doi.org/10.1007/s10940-009-9087-5

Apel, R., & Sweeten, G. (2010). The impact of incarceration on employment during the transition to adulthood. *Social Problems, 57*(3), 448–479. https://doi.org/10.1525/sp.2010.57.3.448

Arditti, J. A., Lambert-Shute, J., & Joest, K. (2003). Saturday morning at the jail: Implications of incarceration for families and children. *Family Relations, 52*(3), 195–204. https://doi.org/10.1111/j.1741-3729.2003.00195.x

Augustine, D., & Kushel, M. (2022). Community supervision, housing insecurity, & homelessness. *The Annals of the American Academy of Political and Social Science, 701*(1), 152–171. https://doi.org/10.1177/00027162221113983

Beckett, K., & Francis, M. M. (2020). The origins of mass incarceration: The racial politics of crime and punishment in the Post-Civil Rights Era. *Annual Review of Law and Social Science, 16*, 433–452. https://doi.org/10.1146/annurev-lawsocsci-110819-100304

Bruns, A. (2019). The third shift: Multiple job holding and the incarceration of women's partners. *Social Science Research, 80*(1), 202–215. https://doi.org/10.1016/j.ssresearch.2018.12.024

Budd, K. (2024). *Incarcerated women and girls*. The Sentencing Project. https://www.sentencingproject.org/fact-sheet/incarcerated-women-and-girls/

Bureau of Justice Administration. (2022). *Violent offender incarceration and truth-in-sentencing incentive formula grant program*. May 17.

Carson, E. A., & Kluckow, R. (2023). *Prisoners in 2022 – statistical tables*. Bureau of Justice Statistics.

Clear, T. R. (2008). The effects of high imprisonment rates on communities. *Crime and Justice, 37*(1), 97–132. https://doi.org/10.1086/522360

Comfort, M. (2008). *Doing time together: Love and family in the shadow of prison*. University of Chicago Press.

Comfort, M., Grinstead, O., McCartney, K., Bourgois, P., & Knight, K. (2005). "You can't do nothing in this damn place": Sex and intimacy among couples with an incarcerated male partner. *Journal of Sex Research, 42*(1), 3–12. https://doi.org/10.1080/00224490509552251

Couloute, L., & Kopf, D. (2018). *Out of prison & out of work: Unemployment among formerly incarcerated people*. Prison Policy Initiative.

Cullen, J. (2018). *Sentencing laws and how they contribute to mass incarceration*. Brennan Center for Justice.

DeHart, D., Shapiro, C., & Clone, S. (2018). "The pill line is longer than the chow line": The impact of incarceration on prisoners and their families. *The Prison Journal, 98*(2), 188–212. https://doi.org/10.1177/0032885517753159

Durante, K. A. (2021). County-level context and sentence lengths for Black, Latinx, and white individuals sentenced to prison: A multi-level assessment. *Criminal Justice Policy Review, 32*(9), 915–937. https:// https://doi.org/10.1177/08874034211021893

Durante, K. A., Phillips Meertins, J. R., & Tadros, E. (2024). Institutional relational maintenance barriers and perceptions of relationship quality among women with incarcerated partners. *Crime & Delinquency, 70*(3), 788–811. https://doi.org/10.1177/00111287221113304

Durante, K. A., Tadros, E., Braxton, C., & Barbini, M. (2023). Supportive communication skills as a protective factor among couples experiencing incarceration. *Criminal Justice and Behavior, 50*(11), 1643–1660. https://doi.org/10.1177/00938548231195036

Firth, C. L., Maher, J. E., Dilley, J. A., Darnell, A., & Lovrich, N. P. (2019). Did marijuana legalization in Washington State reduce racial disparities in adult marijuana arrests? *Substance Use & Misuse, 54*(9), 1582–1587. https://doi.org/10.1080/10826084.2019.1593007

Freiburger, T. L., Jordan, K. L., & Hilinski-Rosick, C. M. (2019). A multivariate analysis of incarceration and sentence length decisions for older defendants. *Criminal Justice Policy Review, 30*(7), 1064–1085. https://doi.org/10.1177/0887403418765911

Garland, D. (2001). *The culture of control: Crime and social order in contemporary society.* Oxford University Press.

Geller, A., Cooper, C. E., Garfinkel, I., Schwartz-Soicher, O., & Mincy, R. B. (2012). Beyond absenteeism: Father incarceration and child development. *Demography, 49*, 49–76. https://doi.org/10.1007/s13524-011-0081-9

Geller, A., & Franklin, A. W. (2014). Paternal incarceration and the housing security of urban mothers. *Journal of Marriage and the Family, 76*(2), 411–427. https://doi.org/10.1111/jomf.12098

Geller, A., Garfinkel, I., Cooper, C. E., & Mincy, R. B. (2009). Parental incarceration and child well-being: Implications for urban families. *Social Science Quarterly, 90*(5), 1186–1202. https://doi.org/10.1111/j.1540-6237.2009.00653.x

Ghandnoosh, N., Barry, C., & Trinka, L. (2023). One in Five: Racial disparity in imprisonment – causes and remedies. *The Sentencing Project.* https://www.sentencingproject.org/reports/one-in-five-racial-disparity-in-imprisonment-causes-and-remedies/

Gordon, G., Jones, J. B., Neelakantan, U., & Athreya, K. (2023). Incarceration, employment, and earnings: Dynamics and differences. *Review of Economic Dynamics, 51*, 677–697. https://doi.org/10.1016/j.red.2023.06.007

Hagan, J. (2010). *Who are the criminals? The politics of crime policy from the age of Roosevelt to the age of Reagan.* Princeton University Press.

Harcourt, K. T., Adler-Baeder, F., Rauer, A., Pettit, G. S., & Erath, S. (2017). Relationship education for incarcerated adults. *Family Process, 56*(1), 75–90. https://doi.org/10.1111/famp.12164

Harman, J. J., Smith, V. E., & Egan, L. C. (2007). The impact of incarceration on intimate relationships. *Criminal Justice and Behavior, 34*(6), 794–815. https://doi.org/10.1177/0093854807299543

Herbert, C. W., Morenoff, J. D., & Harding, D. J. (2015). Homelessness and housing insecurity among former prisoners. *The Russell Sage Foundation Journal of the Social Sciences, 1*(2), 44–79. https://doi.org/10.7758/rsf.2015.1.2.04

Hinton, E. (2020). From the war on poverty to the war on crime: The making of mass incarceration in America (2016). In D. B. Corey Walker & Aimee Meredith Cox (Eds.), *Racism in America: A reader* (pp. 98–106). Harvard University Press. https://doi.org/10.4159/9780674251656-013

Horton, K. B. (2023). An overview of parental incarceration in African American students: The effects on socioeconomics, educational outcomes, school exclusion, and juvenile justice involvement. *Journal of Child & Adolescent Trauma, 16*, 259–267. https://doi.org/10.1007/s40653-022-00504-y

Houle, B. (2014). The effect of incarceration on adult male BMI trajectories, USA, 1981–2006. *Journal of Racial and Ethnic Health Disparities, 1*(1), 21–28. https://doi.org/10.1007/s40615-013-00031

Huebner, B. M. (2005). The effect of incarceration on marriage and work over the life course. *Justice Quarterly, 22*(3), 281–303. https://doi.org/10.1080/07418820500089141

Jahn, J. L., Chen, J. T., Agénor, A., & Krieger, N. (2020). County-level jail incarceration and preterm birth among non-Hispanic Black and white U.S. women, 1999–2015. *Social Science & Medicine*, 112856. https://doi.org/10.1016/j.socscimed.2020.112856

Jordan, K. L., & Freiburger, T. L. (2015). The effect of race/ethnicity on sentencing: Examining sentence type, jail length, and prison length. *Journal of Ethnicity in Criminal Justice, 13*(3), 179–196. https://doi.org/10.1080/15377938.2014.984045

Kluckow, R., & Zeng, Z. (2022). *Correctional populations in the United States, 2020 – statistical tables.* Bureau of Justice Statistics.

Kouyoumdjian, F. G., Kiefer, L., Wobeser, W., Gonzalez, A., & Hwang, S. W. (2016). Mortality over 12 years of follow-up in people admitted to provincial custody in Ontario: A retrospective cohort study. *CMAJ Open, 4*(2), E153–E161. https://doi.org/10.9778/cmajo.20150098

Krivo, L. J., Lyons, C. J., & Vélez, M. B. (2021). The U.S. racial structure and ethno-racial inequality in urban neighborhood crime, 2010–2013. *Sociology of Race and Ethnicity, 7*(3), 350–368. https://doi.org/10.1177/2332649220948551

Latham-Mintus, K., Deck, M. M., & Nelson, E. (2023). Aging with incarceration histories: An intersectional examination of incarceration and health outcomes among older adults. *The Journals of Gerontology: Series B, 78*(5), 853–865. https://doi.org/10.1093/geronb/gbac088

Lee, H., Wildeman, C., Wang, E. A., Matusko, N., & Jackson, J. S. (2014). A heavy burden: The cardiovascular health consequences of having a family member incarcerated. *American Journal of Public Health, 104*(3), 421–427. https://doi.org/10.2105/AJPH.2013.301504

Liedka, R. V., Piehl, A. M., & Useem, B. (2006). The crime-control effect of incarceration: Does scale matter? *Criminology & Public Policy, 5*(2), 245–276. https://doi.org/10.1111/j.1745-9133.2006.00376.x

Liem, M., & Kunst, M. (2013). Is there a recognizable post-incarceration syndrome among released "lifers"? *International Journal of Law and Psychiatry, 36*(3), 333–337. https://doi.org/10.1016/j.ijlp.2013.04.012

Martinez, B. P., Petersen, N., & Omori, M. (2020). Time, money, and punishment: Institutional racial-ethnic inequalities in pretrial detention and case outcomes. *Crime & Delinquency, 66*(6), 837–863. https:// doi.org/10.1177/00111 28719 881600

Massey, D. S. (2016). Segregation and the perpetuation of disadvantage. In D. Brady & L. Burton's (Eds.), *The Oxford handbook of the social science of poverty* (pp. 369–393). Oxford University Press.

Massoglia, M. (2008). Incarceration as exposure: The prison, infectious disease, and other stress-related illnesses. *Journal of Health and Social Behavior, 49*(1), 56–71. https://doi.org/10.1177/002214650804900105

McLeod, B. A., Johnson Jr., W. E., Cryer-Coupet, Q., & Mincy, R. B. (2019). Examining the longitudinal effects of paternal incarceration and coparenting relationships on sons' educational outcomes: A mediation analysis. *Children and Youth Services Review, 100*, 362–375. https://doi.org/10.1016/j.childyouth.2019.03.010

National Research Council and Institute of Medicine. (2013). *Health and incarceration: A workshop summary*. The National Academies Press.

Nellis, A. (2024). *Mass incarceration trends*. The Sentencing Project.

Nicosia, N., Macdonald, J. M., & Arkes, J. (2013). Disparities in criminal court referrals to drug treatment and prison for minority men. *American Journal of Public Health, 103*(6), e77–e84. https://doi.org/10.2105/AJPH.2013.301222

Ofer, U. (2019). *How the 1994 Crime Bill fed the mass incarceration crisis*. American Civil Liberties Union.

Pager, D., Western, B., & Bonikowski, B. (2009). Discrimination in a low-wage labor market: A field experiment. *American Sociological Review, 74*(5), 777–799. https://doi.org/10.1177/000312240907400505

Pfaff, J. F. (2017). *Locked in: The true causes of mass incarceration—and how to achieve real reform*. Basic Books.

Piper, A., & Berle, D. (2019). The association between trauma experienced during incarceration and PTSD outcomes: A systematic review and meta-analysis. *The Journal of Forensic Psychiatry & Psychology, 30*(5), 854–875. https://doi.org/10.1080/14789949.2019.1639788

Porter, L., & DeMarco, L. M. (2018). Beyond the dichotomy: Incarceration dosage and mental health. *Criminology, 57*(1), 136–156. https://doi.org/10.1111/1745-9125.12199

Pratt, D., Piper, M., Appleby, L., Webb, R., & Shaw, J. (2006). Suicide in recently released prisoners: A population-based cohort study. *Lancet, 368*(9530), 119–123. https://doi.org/10.1016/S0140-6736(06)69002-8

Prison Policy Initiative. (2024). *Native incarceration in the U.S.*

Provencher, A., & Conway, J. M. (2019). Health effects of family member incarceration in the United States: A meta-analysis and cost study. *Children and Youth Services Review, 103*, 87–89. https://doi.org/10.1016/j.childyouth.2019.05.029

Redburn, S., Western, B., & Travis, J. (2014). *The growth of incarceration in the United States: Exploring causes and consequences*. National Academies Press.

Robey, J. P., Massoglia, M., & Light, M. T. (2023). A generational shift: Race and the declining lifetime risk of imprisonment. *Demography, 60*(4), 977–1003. https://doi.org/10.1215/00703370-10863378

Roddy, A. L., & Durante, K. A. (2024). Race, perceived neighborhood characteristics, and post-release employability among incarcerated men. *Crime & Delinquency*. Advanced online publication. https://doi.org/10.1177/00111287241264270

Rogers, S. M., Khan, M. R., Tan, S., Turner, C. F., Miller, W. C., & Erbelding, E. (2012). Incarceration, high-risk sexual partnerships, and sexually transmitted infections in an urban population. *Sexually Transmitted Infections, 88*(1), 63–68. https://doi.org/10.1136/sextrans-2011-050280

Rosen, D. L., Wohl, D. A., & Schoenbach, V. J. (2011). All-cause and cause-specific mortality among black and white North Carolina state prisoners, 1995–2005. *Annals of Epidemiology, 21*(10), 719–726. https://doi.org/10.1016/j.annepidem.2011.04.007

Rovner, J. (2023a). Black disparities in youth incarceration. *The Sentencing Project*. https://www.sentencingproject.org/reports/black-disparities-in-youth-incarceration/

Rovner, J. (2023b). Latinx disparities in youth incarceration. *The Sentencing Project*. https://www.sentencingproject.org/reports/latinx-disparities-in-youth-incarceration/

Sampson, R. J., & Loeffler, C. (2010). Punishment's place: The local concentration of mass incarceration. *Daedalus, 139*(3), 20–31.

Saunders, V. (2018). What does your dad do for a living? Children of prisoners and their experiences of stigma. *Children and Youth Services Review, 90*, 21–27. https://doi.org/10.1016/j.childyouth.2018.05.012

Schnittker, J., Massoglia, M., & Uggen, C. (2012). Out and down: Incarceration and psychiatric disorders. *Journal of Health and Social Behavior, 53*(4), 448–464. https://doi.org/10.1177/0022146512453928

Siennick, S. E., Stewart, E. A., & Staff, J. (2014). Explaining the association between incarceration and divorce. *Criminology, 52*(3), 371–398. https://doi.org/10.1111/1745-9125.12040

Steffensmeier, D., Painter-Davis, N., & Ulmer, J.T. (2017). Intersections of race, ethnicity, gender, and age on criminal punishment. *Sociological Perspectives 60*(4), 810–833. https://doi.org/10.1177/0731121416 679371

Sundaresh, R., Yi, Y., Harvey, T. D., Roy, B., Riley, C., Lee, H., Wildeman, C., & Wang, E. A. (2021). Exposure to family member incarceration and adult well-being in the United States. *JAMA Network Open, 4*(5), e2111821. https://doi.org/10.1001/jamanetworkopen.2021.11821

Swanson, C., Lee, C.-B., Sansone, F. A., & Tatum, K. M. (2013). Incarcerated fathers and their children: Perceptions of barriers to their relationships. *The Prison Journal, 93*(4), 453–474. https://doi.org/10.1177/0032885513501024

Tadros, E., Durante, K. A., McKay, T., Barbini, M., & Hollie, B. (2022). Mental health, perceived consensus of coparenting, and physical health among incarcerated fathers and their nonincarcerated, romantic partners. *Families, Systems, & Health, 40*(2), 210–224. https://doi.org/10.1037/fsh0000671

Tadros, E., Durante, K. A., Morgan, A. A., & Hutcherson, R. (2022). An actor-partner interdependence model analysis of family support and depression among coparenting couples with an incarcerated partner. *Journal of Offender Rehabilitation, 61*(7), 390–410.

Tasca, M. (2016). The gatekeepers of contact: Child–caregiver dyads and parental prison visitation. *Criminal Justice and Behavior, 43*(6), 739–758. https://doi.org/10.1177/0093854815613528

Testa, A., & Jackson, D. B. (2020). Incarceration exposure and maternal food insecurity during pregnancy: Findings from the Pregnancy Risk Assessment Monitoring System (PRAMS), 2004–2015. *Maternal and Child Health Journal, 24*, 54–61. https://doi.org/10.1007/s10995-019-02822-4

The United States Sentencing Commission. (2007). *Report to the Congress: Cocaine and federal sentencing policy*.

Turney, K. (2015). Hopelessly devoted? Relationship quality during and after incarceration. *Journal of Marriage and Family, 77*(2), 480–495. https://doi.org/10.1111/jomf.12174

Turney, K. (2017). The unequal consequences of mass incarceration for children. *Demography, 54*(1), 361–389. https://doi.org/10.1007/s13524-016-0543-1

Turney, K. (2021). Family member incarceration and mental health: Results from a nationally representative survey. SSM – *Mental Health, 1*, 100002. https://doi.org/10.1016/j.ssmmh.2021.100002

Uggen, C., Larson, R., Shannon, S., Stewart, R., & Hauf, M. (2024). *Locked out 2024: Four million denied voting rights due to a felony conviction*. The Sentencing Project. Vera Institute of Justice. (2024). *Mass incarceration in numbers.*

Vieraitis, L. M., Kovandzic, T. V., & Marvell, T. B. (2007). The criminogenic effects of imprisonment: Evidence from state panel data, 1974–2002. *Criminology & Public Policy, 6*(3), 589–622. https://doi.org/10.1111/j.1745-9133.2007.00456.x

Wacquant, L. (2010). Class, race & hyperincarceration in revanchist America. *Daedalus, 139*(3), 74–90.

Wang, E. A., Pletcher, M., Lin, F., Vittinghoff, E., Kertesz, S. G., Kiefe, C. I., & Bibbins-Domingo, K. (2009). Incarceration, incident hypertension, and access to health care: Findings from the coronary artery risk development in young adults (CARDIA) study. *Archives of Internal Medicine, 169*(7), 687–693.

Western, B., Kling, J. R., & Weiman, D. F. (2001). The labor market consequences of incarceration. *Crime & Delinquency, 47*(3), 410–427. https://doi.org/10.1177/0011128701047003007

Western, B., & Pettit, B. (2010). Incarceration & social inequality. *Daedalus, 139*(3), 8–19.

Wildeman, C., Lee, H., & Comfort, M. (2013). A new vulnerable population? The health of female partners of men recently released from prison. *Women's Health Issues, 23*(6), e335–e340. https://doi.org/10.1016/j.whi.2013.07.006

Wildeman, C., Schnittker, J., & Turney, K. (2012). Despair by association? The mental health of mothers with children by recently incarcerated fathers. *American Sociological Review, 77*(2), 216–243. https://doi.org/10.1177/0003122411436234

Wooldredge, J., Frank, J., Goulette, N., & Lawrence, I. I. I. T. (2015). Is the impact of cumulative disadvantage on sentencing greater for Black defendants? *Criminology & Public Policy, 14*(2), 182–223. https://doi.org/10.1111/1745-9133.12124

Wu, G., Durante, K. A., & Melton, H. (2024). Pipe dreams: Cannabis legalization and the persistence of racial disparities in jail incarceration. *Journal of Criminal Justice*, 102230. https://doi.org/10.1016/j.jcrimjus.2024.102230

Wu, G., Durante, K. A., Melton, H. C., & Roddy, A. L. (2023). Marijuana legalization and racial disparities in prison incarceration in Colorado and Washington State: A quasi-experimental study. *Journal of Experimental Criminology, 21*, 325–348. https://doi.org/10.1007/s11292-023-09590-w

Chapter 3

Incarcerated Parent-Child Relationships

Eunice Gomez and Eman Tadros

Overview of Incarceration Trends and Rates

The United States (U.S.) presently incarcerates its citizens at exceptionally high rates compared to other countries. Between 1991 and 2007, the number of incarcerated parents in state and federal prisons rose by 79%, or 357,300 parents (Glaze & Maruschak, 2010). Further, in the US, the majority of incarcerations occur in jails, which are operated by local governments or sheriffs' offices and house individuals serving misdemeanor sentences or those detained while awaiting charges, conviction, or sentencing. This is in contrast to prisons, which are run by state or federal governments and house individuals with felony convictions who often serve sentences of more than a year (Sawyer & Wagner, 2020). These kinds of incarceration differ significantly in terms of child development (Turney & Conner, 2019). These differences include the amount of time individuals spend in correctional facilities, the variety and nature of educational and treatment programs available, the proximity of these facilities to where their families live, and the types and frequency of family visits (Shlafer et al., 2015).

Incarcerated Parent-Child Relationships

Parental incarceration is no longer an uncommon adverse childhood event in the United States, since incarceration rates have skyrocketed over the last 50 years. Approximately 2.6 million children in the US today have a parent in jail or prison (Sykes & Pettit, 2014) and the majority of incarcerated individuals have children under the age of 18 (Murphey & Cooper, 2015). A child with an incarcerated parent is deemed high-risk and is more likely to exhibit behavioral problems, mental health issues, and delinquency than a child with non-incarcerated parents (Reho et al., 2021). Children with incarcerated parents frequently face more adversity than their peers, such as the dissolution of marriages or relationships between parents, parents' substance abuse, extreme poverty, residential instability, and homelessness

DOI: 10.4324/9781003542940-3

(Wakefield & Wildeman, 2013), making it critical to consider factors that differentiate families prior to incarceration. To highlight the prevalence of having a family member who is incarcerated, particularly a parent, Sesame Street created Alex in 2013, making him the show's first character with an incarcerated father (Poehlmann-Tynan & Turney, 2021).

Fathers make up the majority of incarcerated parents, with over 57% of men in federal prisons and 46% of men in state prisons having minor children (Maruschak et al., 2021). Paternal incarceration puts a strain on family members, who must navigate institutional barriers to maintain contact with the incarcerated individual. In the absence of the incarcerated parent, families face an array of new stressors, including loss of income, reduced social support, and the absence of an emotional and physical coparenting partner, demonstrating the multifaceted effects of incarceration on families (DeHart et al., 2018). These effects are not equally distributed throughout society at large. Rather, families of color are affected disproportionately (Elderbroom et al., 2018). Although fathers are far more likely to be incarcerated than mothers, maternal and paternal incarceration differ in ways that may have varying effects on children's well-being (Dallaire, 2007). Mothers are more likely than fathers to have lived with their children before being incarcerated, as well as to report adverse experiences, mental health issues, and substance abuse, all of which can have an impact on parenting. Furthermore, children with incarcerated mothers face higher risks on average than those with incarcerated fathers, including a larger possibility of being placed in foster care (Dallaire, 2007). The vast majority of the research on the familial effects of incarceration is focused on incarcerated male family members (e.g., sons and fathers) as well as parental incarceration rather than justice-involved children, despite the fact that almost 13% of U.S. parents have a child in the system (Elderbroom et al., 2018).

Parental Incarceration and Child Risk Factors

Although each case is unique, and each child responds differently, research has shown that a parent's incarceration poses a number of risks to a child's emotional, physical, educational, and economic well-being. Specifically, children of an incarcerated parent are most at risk for developing behavioral and social-emotional issues (Provenchera & Conway, 2019; Turney & Halpern-Meekin, 2020). Further, children with incarcerated parents often face disruptions in their living arrangements, while their caregivers are at higher risk of engaging in delinquency, antisocial behavior, and future incarceration as well as negative physical and mental health outcomes, including heightened health issues, academic struggles, and antisocial behaviors (Beckmeyer & Arditti, 2014). Moreover, they are more prone to developing mental illnesses such as depression and anxiety compared to peers whose parents are not involved in the criminal justice system (Kitzmiller et al., 2021). This adverse childhood experience significantly increases their vulnerability to psychological distress (Gifford et al., 2019). However, family members can mitigate some of these effects by responding to children's emotional needs with empathy, sensitivity, and support (Poehlmann-Tynan et al., 2017). Schools also play a key role in reducing negative outcomes by offering emotional counseling services (Finkeldey & Dennison, 2020), highlighting the importance of emotional intelligence and meaningful connections when supporting children with incarcerated parents.

Psychological/Emotional

Adverse childhood experiences can increase the likelihood of psychological distress (Gifford et al., 2019). Children of incarcerated parents may develop internalized feelings of guilt over their parents' crimes. They may also be concerned about being associated with the offending parent, as this could cause them to be viewed negatively. Further, infants may be fussier than usual depending on how much contact they had with the incarcerated parent prior to incarceration (Schramm & Pucci, 2016). Many young children, toddlers, preschoolers, and school-age children experience sadness, confusion, guilt, abandonment, and anxiety about their relationship with the absent parent (Herreros-Fraile et al., 2023). They may experience separation anxiety and blame themselves for their parent's absence, resulting in negative behaviors such as bedwetting, nightmares, sleeping issues, loss of appetite, and tantrums (Schramm & Pucci, 2016). Preteens and teenagers also may experience comparable ostracism or discrimination from their classmates. To avoid rejection or embarrassment children may isolate themselves from their incarcerated parent, fearing that they, too, might find themselves in prison (Herreros-Fraile et al., 2023).

Physical

Poor physical health is a major concern for children aged 0 to 6, even more so than later in development. Research has also found a relationship between parental incarceration and poor physical health in children (Austin et al., 2022). This emphasizes the significance of addressing physical health concerns throughout early childhood, since they can have implications for overall well-being and development. For instance, Sykes and Pettit (2015), state that children under the age of 18 with unmet and delayed health needs were twice as likely to have a parent who had been incarcerated. Similarly, Turney (2018) found that children who experienced parental incarceration were 1.26x as likely to have unmet healthcare needs. These findings emphasize the significant impact of parental incarceration on children's access to healthcare. Further research has found that children exposed to parental incarceration have shorter sleep durations and demonstrate poor eating habits such as higher fast-food consumption and lower intake of fruits and vegetables than children who are not exposed (Hiolski et al., 2019).

Additionally, in a prospective cohort study of 58,848 Danish citizens born in 1991, Wildeman et al. (2014) found that boys with an incarcerated father were twice as likely to die before the age of 19 compared to boys without an incarcerated father. This pattern was not observed in girls, and mother incarceration did not significantly predict mortality in either boys or girls. The data indicate that both child and parent gender may influence the association between parental incarceration and child health. Also, Lee et al. (2013) examined the impacts of mother and father incarceration on health outcomes and discovered that paternal incarceration had the most significant impact. A father's incarceration history was associated with a higher risk for developing asthma, migraines, high cholesterol, and reporting fair or poor health, as well as a fourfold increase in the risk of HIV/AIDS. However, paternal incarceration was not associated with a higher risk of cancer, hypertension, diabetes, heart disease, or hepatitis. In contrast, maternal incarceration had no significant association with physical health outcomes.

Moreover, the most common health-risk behaviors in adolescents consisted of substance misuse and sexual behavior. Previous studies on adolescent sexual behavior have also found a connection between the early onset of sexual relationships and sexual risks (Luk et al., 2023). Furthermore, past studies have established a significant association between parental incarceration and substance misuse (alcohol, tobacco, drugs, marijuana, etc.) (Whitten et al., 2019).

Behavioral

Some of the most prevalent outcomes considered in research on children with incarcerated fathers and mothers are behavior problems, mental health challenges, and delinquency (Poehlmann-Tynan, & Turney, 2021). Paternal incarceration is associated with additional behavioral issues in nine-year-olds, including attention deficits, internalizing behaviors such as withdrawal and anxiety, and self-reported delinquency (Turney & Goodsell, 2018). Further, Domżalska et al. (2022) found that sons of incarcerated fathers had higher levels of thought and attention problems, whereas daughters had higher levels of attention problems, delinquent and aggressive behavior, externalizing issues, and general behavioral disorders. This suggests that daughters may be more profoundly affected by their fathers' absence, with heightened difficulties in five areas, including the total behavior problems score (Domżalska et al., 2022).

Child Criminal Involvement

There is a concern that if a parent is incarcerated, it might lead to their children and future generations also getting involved in criminal activity. The challenges and stigma associated with parental incarceration are exacerbated in families with an imprisoned female member, particularly mothers. A survey of 6,146 incarcerated individuals in state and federal correctional facilities found that if a parent is incarcerated, a child is six times more likely to be incarcerated, with mothers 2.5 times more likely than fathers to report that their adult children are incarcerated (Dallaire, 2007). Additionally, in a longitudinal study of 5,873 youth, Chavira and colleagues (2017) found that adult children of incarcerated mothers are 75% more likely to be convicted of a crime and served probation than those without an incarcerated mother. Furthermore, parental incarceration increases the risk of substance abuse and domestic violence among impacted children (Chavira et al., 2017). Approximately 75% of children with an incarcerated mother experience severe stress, which contributes to poor social-emotional development and mental health (DeHart et al., 2018). These children also perform poorly academically, are more likely to engage in disruptive behavior at school and have a higher dropout rate (Chesney-Lind, 2015). Moreover, female incarceration has a greater impact on offspring rearrest rates than father incarceration (Tasca et al., 2011).

Subsequently, recent research has identified same-sex gender-specific pathways into the criminal justice system, demonstrating that daughters have a higher risk of criminal justice involvement if their mother is incarcerated, compared to sons and incarcerated fathers (Thomson et al., 2020). Incarceration affects not only the person incarcerated, but also their loved ones (Elderbroom et al., 2018). The disruption of the maternal-child relationship has a negative impact on child development, making children more socially and emotionally vulnerable and more likely to become personally involved in the criminal justice system as adults (Belknap & Holsinger, 2006).

Educational/Academic

Turney and Goodsell (2018) found children who are already vulnerable, – meaning they may be facing challenges such as poverty, unstable family environments, mental health issues, or a lack of access to resources – are the most likely to experience a parental incarceration, which leads to a massive threat against four aspects of the child's well-being, one of them being education. Research generally suggests that parental involvement in schooling improves academic achievement and educational attainment, reduces the likelihood of dropout, and minimizes behavioral problems in children at various stages of development (Child Trends, 2013). Children with an incarcerated parent undergo considerable cognitive and educational development from the ages of 0 to 6 (Herreros-Fraile et al., 2023). These children are more likely to have concentration issues (Geller et al., 2011), lack proper academic preparation (Testa & Jackson, 2021), and repeat grades (Turney & Haskins, 2014). This stage is crucial for cognitive development, particularly the attentional filter (Klenberg et al., 2001), which influences academic adaptation to preschool and kindergarten. Given that the early years are critical for acquiring literacy and initial math skills, it is particularly concerning that the most problems occur during this stage, as they can lead to difficulties that last throughout a child's education (Haskins et al., 2018).

Moreover, father incarceration during early or middle childhood is associated with poorer cognitive outcomes for nine-year-old children, such as reduced reading comprehension, math proficiency, and memory skills (Haskins, 2017). Additional evidence indicates that older children of formerly incarcerated fathers have worse educational attainment, lower academic performance, and higher rates of school absenteeism than children whose fathers were never incarcerated (Haskins, 2016). Understanding the connection between families, schools, and the criminal justice system is critical because schools can act as pipelines, providing access to resources and opportunities for economic mobility and integration into society. However, contemporary schools can also serve as surveillance institutions, keeping formal records, improving security measures, and creating direct connections with other public agencies. As a result, parents who are affiliated with, involved with, or fearful of the criminal justice system may disengage from schools, reducing or inhibiting their involvement in their children's education (Haskins & Jacobsen, 2017).

Economic Well-Being

Casey et al. (2015) documented the prevalence of children of incarcerated parents (COIP) among homeless and highly mobile (HHM) families, an intersection that has not previously been examined in the context of families. The findings show a remarkably high co-occurrence, with nearly one-third (32.6%) of HHM children experiencing parental incarceration (Casey et al., 2015). These findings point to a disproportionately high rate of parental incarceration among children experiencing homelessness. Previous research also indicates that homelessness and incarceration often interact, resulting in a recurring cycle. Incarceration raises a person's chances of being homeless (Petersilia, 2001). Limited resources, limited job training, housing restrictions for convicted felons, and the stigma of incarceration often lead many individuals to become homeless shortly after their release (Kushel et al., 2005). Further, parental incarceration also massively strains family life, with cascading consequences for children (Turney & Goodsell,

2018). For example, it increases families' economic hardship. Incarcerated parents, many of whom were helping to support their families financially before their confinement, cannot earn substantial income during incarceration (Turney & Goodsell, 2018). At the same time, they are like to accumulate fines, fees, and legal debts. Upon release, the stigma of a criminal record can make it difficult for them to find work and makes them more likely to avoid mainstream institutions such as banks, hospitals, and schools (Turney & Goodsell, 2018).

Paternal Incarceration, Parenting, and Effects on Children

The nuanced impact of parental incarceration on children can be attributed, in part, to the living situation of the incarcerated parent before imprisonment. Turney and Wildeman (2013) explained that the detrimental effects on parent-child relationships are heightened when the incarcerated parent had been residing with their family prior to incarceration. Turney and Wildeman (2013) observed that the relationships between fathers and children, as well as fathers and mothers, remained unaffected by paternal incarceration when fathers were not residentially connected to their families before entering prison. The connection between a father's parenting behaviors and incarceration is influenced by his relationship with the mother, highlighting how the non-incarcerated parent plays a crucial role in determining the incarcerated parent's ability to maintain a relationship with their children (Turney & Wildeman, 2013).

The family characteristics and processes as well as the child's age inform the relationship between parental incarceration and child development/youth outcomes. Fathers are more likely to be in contact with their younger children (McKay et al., 2018). In summary, the repercussions of parental incarceration reach across multiple dimensions of family life, impacting the incarcerated individual, their partners, children, and external social networks. Coparents face substantial challenges, including financial stress, adjusting to new roles, and overcoming institutional barriers. Social support proves to be a resilient factor for many families coping with the incarceration of a loved one. The living arrangement before incarceration influences the degree of impact on children, particularly those residing with the incarcerated parent. Navigating the intricate terrain of parental incarceration necessitates a comprehensive understanding of socioeconomic factors, cultural contexts, and family characteristics, which are essential for developing targeted interventions.

Parent-Child Communication

Prior research has found that many incarcerated parents report that the hardest part about being incarcerated is the separation from their children (e.g., Poehlmann-Tynan & Pritzl, 2019), and many incarcerated parents report elevated symptoms of depression when they have lower levels of contact with their children (e.g. Poehlmann, 2005). While parent-child visits can be a source of positive connection and resilience for incarcerated parents and their children, visits can also highlight negative emotions like sadness and loss in addition to potentially triggering trauma reactions (e.g., the developmental paradox; Arditti & Salva, 2015).

Moreover, research suggests that maintaining contact with an incarcerated parent can benefit children by allowing them to express feelings of loss (Shlafer et al., 2020). However, contact visits in correctional settings are typically limited to minimal physical interaction, such as brief hugs and kisses at the beginning and end of visits (Shlafer et al., 2020). Correctional facilities focus on "safety and security," frequently overlooking the needs of visitors, particularly family members and children (Poehlmann-Tynan, 2015). The approach to accommodating visitors differs between jails and prisons. Jails, which provide short-term incarceration for individuals awaiting trial or serving short sentences, usually allow visitors behind Plexiglass barriers or by video (Poehlmann-Tynan, 2015). Prisons, which are designed for the long-term incarceration of convicted individuals, are more likely to provide face-to-face contact, while video visits are becoming more common (Poehlmann-Tynan, 2015). While child-friendly contact visits with plenty of physical connection are the most beneficial way for young children to communicate with their incarcerated parents during times of health, there are also effective distant methods for communicating (Skora Horgan & Poehlmann-Tynan, 2020). Traditional forms of mediated communication, such as phone calls and letters, can be challenging for very young children due to their limited cognitive, language, and attention abilities (Skora Horgan & Poehlmann-Tynan, 2020). However, emerging kinds of mediated communication, such as in-home video chats, provide a more accessible and developmentally appropriate option for young children to maintain contact with distant family members, including their incarcerated parents.

Preparing for visits and providing adequate support for children, the incarcerated individual, and their families during and after visits is critical, for maintaining family connections, reducing stress, and promoting the well-being of all involved. Providing child-friendly materials, such as a simple sticker from a corrections officer after going through a metal detector, can help make the experience less intimidating and create positive associations with the visit (Poehlmann-Tynan, 2015). More thorough training for corrections personnel could help them engage positively with families and interact with children in a developmentally appropriate way (Poehlmann-Tynan, 2015). Visitation information should also be presented in a clear, child-friendly format, both at the jail entrance and on the facility's website, including visual aids such as drawings of the visiting room and directions for using listening devices (Poehlmann-Tynan, 2015). Families should be given five-minute warnings before the visit ends to avoid surprises or distress from sudden changes, such as a video monitor turning off or the end of a Plexiglas or face-to-face visit (Poehlmann-Tynan, 2015). Plexiglas visits involve a clear acrylic barrier that is frequently used in institutional or correctional settings to separate visitors and the person they are seeing apart yet enabling them to view and communicate without making physical contact. For non-contact visits, privacy could be improved by placing barriers between video or Plexiglas booths.

Implications/Recommendations

Parental incarceration is more consistently harmful to children in the case of paternal incarceration (Wakefield & Wildeman, 2013) and maternal incarceration (Cho, 2010). Families can help decrease the impact of incarceration-related symptoms on children by demonstrating empathy, sensitivity, and responsiveness to their emotional needs (Poehlmann-Tynan et al., 2017). It has been recommended to assist children and their families to manage stress by addressing and understanding ambiguous loss, improving in-person visitation, increasing social support, and providing coping resources for children and their non-incarcerated caregivers (Arditti, 2016). Schramm and Pucci (2016) recommend that infants and young children follow consistent routines and schedules, including regular visits with their incarcerated parent. Assure children and adolescents that they will always have at least one parent to address their needs. Emphasize that the custodial parent will maintain frequent contact with the incarcerated parent and encourage the children to do the same. Comfort children during visitation, as they may be distressed when separated from their parent; a brief explanation of the security procedures in place will help them understand that these measures keep their parent safe until their next visit (Schramm & Pucci, 2016).

Future Directions

Resources for incarcerated family members can help them adjust to life with an incarcerated loved one, addressing the unique emotions during and after incarceration. Both scenarios present new challenges and require adjustments in all areas of life. Increasing access to relational therapy for families of color dealing with a parent's incarceration and developing culturally relevant treatment approaches for incarcerated coparenting are crucial goals (Tadros & Durante, 2022). Additionally, future research should investigate the effects of incarcerated parent–caregiver coparenting interactions on children's mental health, social competence, happiness, and educational outcomes (Tadros et al., 2021). Future challenges for researchers and policymakers will be to examine the best methods to support caregivers prior to incarceration instead of waiting and relying on visitation and correctional services (McCarthy & Adams, 2019). Racial/ethnic, economic, and geographic diversity, as well as disparities, must be considered for further studies on parental incarceration and child development.

References

Arditti, J. A. (2016). A family stress-proximal process model for understanding the effects of parental incarceration on children and their families. *Couple and Family Psychology: Research and Practice*, *5*(2), 65.

Arditti, J. A., & Savla, J. (2015). Parental incarceration and child trauma symptoms in single caregiver homes. *Journal of Child and Family Studies*, *24*(3), 551–561. https://doi.org/10.1007/s10826-013-9867-2

Austin, M. K., White, I. I., & Kim, A. W. (2022). Parental incarceration and child physical health outcomes from infancy to adulthood: A critical review and multilevel model of potential pathways. *American Journal of Human Biology*, *34*(5), e23691. https://doi.org/10.1002/ajhb.23691

Beckmeyer, J., & Arditti, J. (2014). Implications of In-Person Visits for Incarcerated Parents' Family Relationships and Parenting Experience. *Journal of Offender Rehabilitation*, *53*(2), 129. https://doi.org/10.1080/10509674.2013.868390

Belknap, J., & Holsinger, K. (2006). The gendered nature of risk factors for delinquency. *Feminist Criminology*, *1*(1), 48–71. https://doi.org/10.1177/1557085105282897

Casey, E. C., Shlafer, R. J., & Masten, A. S. (2015). Parental incarceration as a risk factor for children in homeless families. *Family Relations*, *64*(4), 490–504. https://doi.org/10.1111/fare.12136

Chavira, D., Fowler, P. J., & Jason, L. A. (2018). Parenting and the association between maternal criminal justice involvement and adolescent delinquency. *Children and Youth Services Review*, *87*, 114–122. https://doi.org/10.1016/j.childyouth.2018.02.013

Child Trends. (2013). *Parental involvement in schools*. Child Trends, Inc.

Cho, R. M. (2010). Maternal incarceration and children's adolescent outcomes: Timing and dosage. *Social Service Review*, *84*(2), 257–282. https://doi.org/10.1086/653456

Dallaire, D. H. (2007). Incarcerated mothers and fathers: A comparison of risks for children and families. *Family Relations*, *56*, 440–453. https://doi.org/10.1111/j.1741-3729.2007.00472.x

DeHart, D., Shapiro, C., & Clone, S. (2018). "The Pill Line Is Longer Than the Chow Line": The impact of incarceration on prisoners and their families. *The Prison Journal*, *98*(2), 188–212. https://doi.org/10.1177/0032885517753159

Domżalska, A., Skowroński, B., & Wolańczyk, T. (2022). Behavioral and emotional problems of prisoners' children based on the children's self-report. *International Journal of Environmental Research and Public Health*, *19*(1), 561. https://doi.org/10.3390/ijerph19010561

Elderbroom, B., Bennett, L., Gong, S., Rose, F., & Towns, Z. (2018). *Every second: The impact of the incarceration crisis on America's families*. FWD. us.

Finkeldey, J. G., & Dennison, C. R. (2020). School-based resources as protective factors from the influence of parental incarceration on depressive symptoms. *Social Currents, 7*(5), 402–423. https://doi.org/10.1177/2329496520921844

Geller, A., Garfinkel, I., & Western, B. (2011). Paternal incarceration and support for children in fragile families. *Demography, 48*, 25–47. https://doi.org/10.1007/s13524-010-0009-9

Gifford, E. J., Golonka, M., Kozecke, L. E., et al. (2019). Association of parental incarceration with psychiatric and functional outcomes of young adults. *JAMA Network Open, 2*(8), e1910005. https://doi.org/10.1001/jamanetworkopen.2019.10005

Glaze, L. E., & Maruschak, L. M. (2010). Parents in prison and their minor children: Bureau of Justice Statistics special report. *Bureau of Justice Statistics*. https://bjs.ojp.gov/content/pub/pdf/pptmc.pdf.

Haskins, A. R. (2017). Paternal Incarceration and Schooling Contexts: Intersecting Inequalities of Educational Opportunity. *Annals of the American Academy of Political and Social Science, 674*, 134-162. https://doi.org/10.1177/0002716217732011

Haskins, A. R., & Jacobsen, W. C. (2017). Schools as surveilling institutions? Paternal incarceration, system avoidance, and parental involvement in schooling. *American Sociological Review, 82*(4), 657–684. https://doi.org/10.1177/0003122417706286

Haskins, A. R., Amorim, M., & Mingo, M. (2018). Parental incarceration and child outcomes: Those at risk, evidence of impacts, methodological insights, and areas of future work. *Sociology Compass, 12*(3), e12562. https://doi.org/10.1111/soc4.12562

Herreros-Fraile, A., Carcedo, R. J., Viedma, A., Ramos-Barbero, V., Fernández-Rouco, N., Gomiz-Pascual, P., & Del Val, C. (2023). Parental incarceration, development, and well-being: A developmental systematic review. *International Journal of Environmental Research and Public Health, 20*(4), 3143. https://doi.org/10.3390/ijerph20043143

Hiolski, K., Eisenberg, M. E., & Shlafer, R. J. (2019). Youth self-reported health and their experience of parental incarceration. *Families, Systems, & Health, 37*(1), 38–47. https://doi.org/10.1037/fsh0000381

Kitzmiller, M. K., Cavanagh, C., Frick, P., Steinberg, L., & Cauffman, E. (2020). Parental incarceration and the mental health of youth in the justice system: The moderating role of neighborhood disorder. *Psychology, Public Policy, and Law*. https://doi.org/2443/10.1037/law0000274

Klenberg, L., Korkman, M., & Lahti-Nuuttila, P. (2001). Differential development of attention and executive functions in 3-to 12-year-old Finn ish children. *Developmental Neuropsychology, 20*(1), 407–428. https://doi.org/10.1207/S15326942DN2001_5

Kushel, M. B., Hahn, J. A., Evans, J. L., Bangsberg, D. R., & Moss, A. R. (2005). Revolving doors: Imprisonment among the homeless and marginally housed population. *American Journal of Public Health, 95*(10), 1747–1752. https://doi.org/10.2105/AJPH.2004.059005

Lee, R. D., Fang, X., & Luo, F. (2013). The impact of parental incarceration on the physical and mental health of young adults. *Pediatrics, 131*(4), e1188–e1195. https://doi.org/10.1542/peds.2012-0627

Luk, M. S. K., Hui, C., Tsang, S. K. M., Fung, Y. L., & Chan, C. H. Y. (2023). Physical and psychosocial impacts of parental incarceration on children and adolescents: A systematic review differentiating age of exposure. *Adolescent Research Review, 8*(2), 159–178. https://doi.org/10.1007/s40894-023-00223-0

Maruschak, L. M., Bronson, J., & Alper, M. (2021). Parents in prison and their minor children: Survey of Prison Inmates, 2016 (NCJ 252645). U.S. Department of Justice, Bureau of Justice Statistics. https://bjs.ojp.gov/library/publications/parents-prison-and-their-minor-children-survey-prison-inmates-2016

McCarthy, D., & Adams, M. (2019). Can family–prisoner relationships ever improve during incarceration? Examining the primary caregivers of incarcerated young men. The British Journal of Criminology, 59(2), 378–395. https://doi.org/10.1093/bjc/azy039

McKay, T., Comfort, M., Grove, L., Bir, A., & Lindquist, C. (2018). Whose punishment, whose crime? Understanding parenting and partnership in a time of mass incarceration. *Journal of Offender Rehabilitation, 57*(2), 69–82. https://doi.org/10.1080/10509674.2017.1294640

Murphey, D., & Cooper, P. M. (2015). Parents behind bars: What happens to their children? *Child Trends.* Retrieved from https://www.childtrends.org/wp-content/uploads/2015/10/2015-42ParentsBehindBars.pdf

Petersilia, J. (2001). Prisoner reentry: Public safety and reintegration challenges. *The Prison Journal, 81*(3), 360–375. https://doi.org/10.1177/0032885501081003004

Poehlmann-Tynan, J. (Ed.). (2015). *Children's contact with incarcerated parents: Implications for policy and intervention.* Springer.

Poehlmann, J. (2005). Representations of attachment relationships in children of incarcerated mothers. *Child Development, 76*(3), 679–696. https://doi.org/10.1111/j.1467-8624.2005.00871.x

Poehlmann-Tynan, J., & Pritzl, K. (2019). Parent–child visits when parents are incarcerated in prison or jail. In J. M. Eddy & J. Poehlmann-Tynan (Eds.), *Handbook on children with incarcerated parents: Research, policy, and practice* (pp. 131–147). Springer International Publishing. https://doi.org/10.1007/978-3-030-16707-3_10

Poehlmann-Tynan, J., & Turney, K. (2021). A developmental perspective on children with incarcerated parents. *Child Development Perspectives, 15*(1), 3–11. https://doi.org/10.1111/cdev.12426

Poehlmann-Tynan, J., Burnson, C., Runion, H., & Weymouth, L. A. (2017). Attachment in young children with incarcerated fathers. *Development and Psychopathology, 29*(2), 389–404. https://doi.org/10.1017/S0954579417000079

Provencher, A., & Conway, J. M. (2019). Health effects of family member incarceration in the United States: A meta-analysis and cost study. *Children and Youth Services Review, 103*, 87–99. https://doi.org/10.1016/j.childyouth.2019.06.013

Reho, A., Corsano, P., & Fruggeri, L. (2021). Co-parenting in families with an imprisoned parent: A systematic review. *Ricerche di psicologia, 3*, 1–30. https://doi.org/10.3280/rip2021oa12855

Sawyer, W., & Wagner, P. (2020). *Mass incarceration: The whole pie 2020.* Prison Policy Initiative. Retrieved from https://www.prisonpolicy.org/reports/pie2020.html

Schramm, D., & Pucci, C. (2016). *Parenting from prison: A co-parenting guide for divorced and separated parents.* University of Missouri Extension. Retrieved from https://extension.missouri.edu/publications/gh6615

Shlafer, R. J., Davis, L., Hindt, L., Weymouth, L., Runion, H., Burnson, C., & Poehlmann-Tynan, J. (2020). Fathers in jail and their minor children: Paternal characteristics

and associations with father-child contact. *Journal of Child and Family Studies, 29*(3), 791–801. https://doi.org/10.1007/s10826-020-01696-3
Shlafer, R. J., Loper, A. B., & Schillmoeller, L. (2015). Introduction and literature review: Is parent–child contact during parental incarceration beneficial? In J. Poehlmann (Ed.), *Children's contact with incarcerated parents* (pp. 1–21). Springer. https://doi.org/10.1007/978-3-319-16625-4_1
Skora Horgan, E., & Poehlmann-Tynan, J. (2020). In-home video chat for young children and their incarcerated parents. *Journal of Children and Media, 14*(3), 400–406. https://doi.org/10.1080/17482798.2020.1758729
Sykes, B. L., & Pettit, B. (2014). Mass incarceration, family complexity, and the reproduction of childhood disadvantage. *The Annals of the American Academy of Political and Social Science, 654*, 127–149. https://doi.org/10.1177/0002716214526345
Sykes, B. L., & Pettit, B. (2015). Severe deprivation and system inclusion among children of incarcerated parents in the United States after the Great Recession. *RSF: The Russell Sage Foundation Journal of the Social Sciences, 1*(2), 108–132. https://doi.org/10.7758/RSF.2015.1.2.05
Tadros, E., & Durante, K. A. (2022). Coparenting, negative educational outcomes, and familial instability in justice-involved families. *International Journal of Offender Therapy and Comparative Criminology, 66*(2), 267–287. https://doi.org/10.1177/0306624X211013740
Tadros, E., Fanning, K., Jensen, S., & Poehlmann-Tynan, J. (2021). Coparenting and mental health in families with jailed parents. *International Journal of Environmental Research and Public Health, 18*(16), 8705. https://doi.org/10.3390/ijerph18168705
Tasca, M., Rodriguez, N., & Zatz, M. S. (2011). Family and Residential Instability in the Context of Paternal and Maternal Incarceration. *Criminal Justice and Behavior, 38*(3), 231–247. https://doi.org/10.1177/0093854810391632
Testa, A., & Jackson, D. B. (2021). Parental incarceration and school readiness: Findings from the 2016 to 2018 National Survey of Children's Health. *Academic Pediatrics, 21*(3), 534–541. https://doi.org/10.1016/j.acap.2020.08.016
Thomson, N. D., Moeller, F. G., Amstadter, A. B., Svikis, D., Perera, R. A., & Bjork, J. M. (2020). The impact of parental incarceration on psychopathy, crime, and prison violence in women. *International Journal of Offender Therapy and Comparative Criminology, 64*(10–11), 1178–1194. https://doi.org/10.1177/0306624X20904695
Turney, K. (2018). Adverse childhood experiences among children of incarcerated parents. *Children and Youth Services Review, 89*, 218–225.
Turney, K., & Conner, E. (2019). Jail incarceration: A common and consequential form of criminal justice contact. *Annual Review of Criminology, 2*, 265–290. https://doi.org/10.1146/annurev-criminol-011518-024601
Turney, K., & Goodsell, R. (2018). Parental incarceration and children's well-being. *The Future of Children, 28*(1), 147–164. https://doi.org/10.1353/foc.2018.0007
Turney, K., & Halpern-Meekin, S. (2020). Parental relationship churning and adolescent well-being: examining instability within families. *Journal of Marriage and Family*. https://doi.org/10.1111/jomf.12665

Turney, K., & Wildeman, C. (2013). Redefining Relationships: Explaining the Countervailing Consequences of Paternal Incarceration for Parenting. *American Sociological Review, 78*(6), 949–979. https://doi.org/10.1177/0003122413505589

Turney, K. & Haskins, A. R. (2014). Falling behind? Children's early grade retention after paternal incarceration. *Sociology of Education 87*, 241–258. https://doi.org/10.1177%2F0038040714547086

Wakefield, S., & Wildeman, C. (2013). *Children of the prison boom: Mass incarceration and the future of American inequality*. Oxford University Press.

Whitten, T., Burton, M., Tzoumakis, S., & Dean, K. (2019). Parental offending and child physical health, mental health, and drug use outcomes: A systematic literature review. *Journal of Child and Family Studies, 28*, 1155–1168. https://doi.org/10.1007/s10826-019-01388-7

Wildeman, C. (2014). Parental incarceration, child homelessness, and the invisible consequences of mass imprisonment. *The Annals of the American Academy of Political and Social Science, 651*(1), 74–96. https://doi.org/10.1177/0002716213502921

Chapter 4

Romantic Relationships Impacted by Incarceration

Intimacy Amidst Isolation

Anna Katherine Waters, Eman Tadros and Maxine Notice

When a romantic partner is incarcerated, it can lead to significant challenges such as financial instability, emotional distress, mental and physical health issues, and parenting difficulties (Arditti et al., 2003; Turney, 2015). The loss of income for the household following incarceration may necessitate reliance on public assistance or require partners of the incarcerated person to take on multiple jobs (Bruns, 2019). Incarceration also introduces additional expenses, including costs associated with visitation. For virtual visitation, families must pay for various communication platforms (Charles et al., 2021). Additionally, money that would typically support the household is now redirected to support the incarcerated individual (Bruns, 2019). Beyond financial challenges, the incarceration of a partner can bring significant emotional strain, particularly for partners, as someone in the family must step in to fill the gap left by the incarcerated individual, demonstrating how incarceration requires family to shift or renegotiate roles due (Arditti, 2003; Tadros & Finney, 2018).

Incarceration has detrimental effects on the mental and physical health of family members. Both children and adults with an incarcerated family member experience poorer health outcomes, with associated costs exceeding $22 billion for adults and $340 million for children (Provencher & Conway, 2019). Furthermore, the health of non-incarcerated family members often deteriorates as a result of additional stress and role strain (Bruns, 2019; Tadros et al., 2022a). They may develop stress-related health conditions, including weakened immune systems, diabetes, high blood pressure, and an increased risk of coronary heart disease (Sumra & Schillaci, 2015).

Incarceration forces isolation, distance, uncertainty, violence, instability, and chaos upon couples and families. During incarceration, partner interactions are sparse and occur within highly surveilled and depressing environments (DeHart et al., 2018). The strengths and challenges of a couple play a critical role in the trajectory of their relationship, especially when couples are also experiencing tremendous stress outside of their relationship (Dwyer

DOI: 10.4324/9781003542940-4

Emory, 2022). According to Durante et al. (2023), couples in which the incarcerated male partner and his female partner resolved conflicts effectively reported higher relationship quality, while those with frequent heated arguments or interruptions were more likely to separate.

Partners of Incarcerated Individuals

Romantic relationships may play a role in reducing recidivism. Marriage is associated with lower criminal activity in what is described as "the marriage effect" (Skardhamar et al., 2015). Previous research has also shown evidence for quality marital and non-marital relationships being protective factors against recidivism (Simons & Barr, 2014). Moreover, Wallace et al. (2020) discovered that a higher quality of romantic relationships was associated with a lower likelihood of reincarceration, surprisingly, in contrast to prior research, being in a romantic relationship was correlated with a higher probability of reincarceration.

Romantic partners and coparents of incarcerated men experience tremendous strain throughout the incarceration period as this separation takes a toll on the quality of their interactions, the coparenting dynamic, parenting, and economic well-being. Those left behind often struggle with emotional and mental health issues such as depression or anxiety, exacerbated by external stressors such as physical separation and financial instability (Yeboaa et al., 2022). Many also carry a sense of shame about their situation, leading them to conceal incarceration, which can result in social isolation and increased depression (Wildeman & Western, 2010).

Instability in the Partner Relationship

Incarceration has been linked to higher divorce rates (Skipper et al., 2020). Stability in couples may stem from responsive parenting in childhood, as secure attachment in incarcerated–non-incarcerated partnerships was associated with stable, sensitive upbringings (Tadros & Ansell, 2022). Higher dyadic adjustment was also linked to lower relationship conflict in these couples (Tadros & Vlach, 2023). Partner dynamics influence family outcomes; in incarcerated couples, parental conflict was associated with children's internalizing and externalizing behaviors (Pech et al., 2020).

Maintaining a relationship during incarceration requires skills for positive, bonding interactions. Not everyone has the privilege of developing these skills early, often due to factors beyond a family's control, such as limited time together or chronic stress. In this way, without intervention, one's level of privilege may affect the stability and cordiality within one's relationship (Tadros et al., 2022b, 2023). Family therapists can help couples build these abilities through compassion, awareness, communication training, and self-regulation tools. For couples facing incarceration, such skills are critical, as each interaction carries heightened stakes for their family, finances, and well-being.

Previous research has shown a connection between maternal parenting stress and child externalizing behaviors (Antle et al., 2019). Furthermore, Turney & Wildeman (2013) indicate a connection between recent paternal incarceration and mothers seeking new partnerships. Considering the elevated parenting stress associated with paternal incarceration, the choice of mothers to re-partner may have a dual effect on the family. On one hand, it can bring relief by introducing additional financial and social support for mothers and children. On the other hand, this repartnering introduces complexities into family life (Turney & Wildeman, 2013).

The distance created by incarceration puts stress on romantic relationships and can lead to suspicion, jealousy, and concerns regarding infidelity that degrade the trust and stability of relationships (Davey-Rothwell et al., 2012). A lack of trust can lead to damaging behavior. For example, distrustful partners may be hostile, controlling, or make hurtful accusations against their partner. Moreover, one's reactivity in their relationship may be made worse by the stress and isolation that is inherent with incarceration.

Daily Challenges

Partners of incarcerated individuals must overcome institutional barriers to maintain ties such as costly phone calls and visits, distance to the facility, and scheduling issues (DeHart et al., 2018; McKay et al., 2018). DeHart et al. (2018) explored female partners of incarcerated fathers disclosed not wanting to expose children to the unpleasantness of the incarceration environment, pointing to how coparenting partners determine the access to communication the incarcerated individual has with children. Overcoming these barriers is exacerbated by the loss of income and parental support from the incarcerated person (McKay et al., 2018). Limited, structured contact can strain families seeking emotional closeness (Tadros et al., 2022c). Families may withhold exchanging information about their lives in an attempt to protect one another from unpleasant experiences in the incarcerated setting or in the outside world (DeHart et al., 2018). Limited time to communicate also complicates relational maintenance (Tadros et al., 2022c). Difficulties include not having enough time to resolve problems, relying on the incarcerated person to make phone contact, and the limited duration of communication inhibiting relationship building/development (Tadros et al., 2022c).

Relationship Strain

The loss of an incarcerated partner often forces the remaining partner to seek additional employment, especially when they previously relied on that person's income (Bruns, 2019). Balancing multiple jobs with household and parenting responsibilities can create extreme role strain, leading some to seek support through repartnering, which can also meet emotional and physical needs (Cooper et al., 2015; Dwyer Emory, 2022). In one study, two-thirds repartnered despite having children, cohabiting, and reporting high relationship quality before incarceration (Dwyer Emory, 2022). While ending a relationship may result in more complicated coparenting or a loss of contact between the incarcerated parent and child, benefits can include relief from strain, new partnership opportunities, or leaving a negative or violent relationship. Women were more likely to remain if partners showed greater romantic support, parental cooperation, less violence, and lower substance use or criminal justice involvement (Dwyer Emory, 2022).

Mothers left behind experience lower support in the absence of their partner report overall decreases in relationship quality and satisfaction (Turney, 2015). There is evidence that romantic partners also experience detrimental effects on emotional and mental health. Physical symptoms are then exacerbated by a barrage of external stressors, including being physically distant from the loved one and shouldering financial burdens (Yeboaa et al., 2022).

Case Application

This case application is a fictional depiction of treatment within a prison: Daryl, an incarcerated individual; Tanya, partner to Daryl; and Sean, the therapist. This case will be explored through a socially and culturally attuned lens, using contextual family therapy.

Daryl is a 24-year-old African American male who has recently been incarcerated in the state of Mississippi. Daryl was convicted of second-degree burglary earlier in the year, as he unlawfully entered and attempted to secure his final check that was being withheld from his last place of employment. Daryl has a forensic history and was sentenced to 90 days in a juvenile detention center at the age of 16 for causing property damage with a group of his peers. Since his detention as a youth, Daryl has tried diligently to stay on the straight and narrow. He has been experiencing excessive guilt over his current sentence of three years, which has led to a mild depressive episode.

Tanya, a 23-year-old Caucasian female, is Daryl's partner and strongest support system member. Tanya and Daryl met in high school and have been in a committed relationship for a year and a half. After beginning their relationship, Daryl moved into Tanya's apartment, seeing it as a way to gain independence from his mother and little sister. Prior to Daryl's incarceration six months ago, the couple enjoyed a connected and passionate relationship, spending time creating art together and enjoying their two rescue dogs.

Sean, a licensed marriage and family therapist (MFT), is a 48-year-old African American male assigned to work with Daryl and Tanya. Sean has been practicing for over ten years professionally and has worked within the prison system for the last six years. Sean has recently been able to advocate for sessions with incarcerated individuals and their system members on a regular basis, through the use of teletherapy technology.

Sean's initial session with Daryl and Tanya consists of completing a biopsychosocial-spiritual intake (Gale, 2022). This acts as a way for him to explore the connections among all facets of the client's life, and account for a variety of areas such as strengths and supports. Both clients grew up just blocks from one another in a low-income housing development. Daryl was raised along with his 12-year-old sister by a single mother who worked as a teacher's aide. Daryl has never known his father and has been historically tasked with being "the man of the house". The role has put him in a position of perpetual thinking of how to protect the women in his life. Daryl noted that this pressure has historically led to moments of him acting out, such as him tagging graffiti and committing vandalism with his peers as a teenager. He feels this was him rebelling against the pressures of adulthood. Daryl notes that he has struggled with making strong friendship connections and has cycled through peers during his time in school and while working. While Daryl was raised within the Christian faith, he notes that he finds himself to be more spiritual as opposed to engaging in organized religion. While he historically considers himself mentally and physically strong, Daryl notes that he has been feeling down on himself for ending up in prison. He never saw himself in this position and is burdened by how it is impacting his life.

Tanya shares that her life has been plagued with hardships, but she has felt she is in a better position in the last few years. She noted that her family has a long history of illegal substance use. Her father was killed due to gun violence while attempting to purchase illegal substances when she was four. Her mother died shortly after due to a drug overdose. After her parents died Tanya was placed in kinship care and raised by her maternal grandmother. Tanya noted that she has always been physically healthy but worked with a therapist throughout grade and middle school to process the loss of her parents. Tanya credits her awareness of the state of her mental health to her years in therapy. She notes that she tries to work diligently to keep a balance of health in her life by taking care of her physical body, her mental wellness, and spiritual engagement through practicing yoga, creating art, and volunteering in her local community. Tanya explains that she has not been able to maintain that balance since Daryl's incarceration.

Sean uses his clinical insight during the intake session to further assess the symptoms the couple are experiencing because of the dramatic shift in their relationship via Daryl's incarceration. Assessments administered include the Generalized Anxiety Disorder Assessment, GAD-7 (Spitzer et al., 2006), which highlights moderate levels of anxiety being experienced by Daryl, and the Patient Health Questionnaire, PHQ-9 (Kroenke & Spitzer, 2002), which highlights a mild level of distress being exhibited by both partners. To further assess the client's current functioning Sean administers a relational inventory, the Dyadic Adjustment Scale (Spanier, 1976). Relationally, while both partners identify a strong commitment to making their relationship work, they also identify barriers of lack of intimacy and being able to confide in one another. Understanding the client's current level of symptom presentation allows Sean the ability to effectively track the couple's experience of symptom relief as they move through the therapy process.

Using a contextual family therapy lens, Sean uses the base tenants of the theory to conceptualize this case. Nagy framed therapy as encompassing four levels: (1) the facts, e.g., the circumstances that impact life experience such as where one is born, key life events such as traumas, losses, and transitions; (2) individual psychology, or the meaning that individuals make of their experience and how that is internalized; (3) transactional patterns involving family communication, structures, and interactions; and (4) relational ethics, fairness in what we give to each other, as the overarching contextual framework for the other dimensions (McDowell et al., 2023).

Extending his clinical practice to one that takes a socioculturally attuned stance while using contextual family therapy, Sean prepares himself to work with the tenants of relational ethics to follow practical steps that address fairness, power, and justice for the client couple. He will use the following practice guidelines as he moves through treatment: (1) Practice Multidirected Sociocultural Attunement; (2) Discuss Sociohistorical Context/Background; (3) Identify and Acknowledge Unfairness; (4) Assume People Want to Give; (5) Encourage Due Crediting; (6) Encourage Accountability; and (7) Focus Forward (McDowell et al., 2023).

While Daryl's incarcerated state is a major focal point in the experience of the couple, Sean uses multidirected sociocultural attunement to allow Tanya's experience to be fully seen and valued within the therapy setting (Sibley et al., 2015). Sean begins his treatment by attending to the facts facing the couple collectively and individually. After the group discusses the impact of Daryl's arrest and incarceration on his depression and isolation, talks move to the role that incarceration has played on the financial burden the couple is experiencing. While Daryl talks about the financial burden limiting his ability to place phone calls to his mother and sister, Sean notices that Tanya remains silent about how the financial hardships have impacted her:

S: We've heard about Daryl's hardships with depression and isolation. On the other side of your relationship, there are your experiences. What has been coming up for you as the most salient areas of concern?

T: For me? I think my health.

S: Your health? Why don't you tell us a bit more about what that looks like for you.

T: Well, I like to make sure that I try to take care of my health by staying balanced as much as I can. But with the current situation things feel out of whack. I mean, I know that things are rough financially so I try to do the best I can by working extra hours. But all the extra work doesn't allow me enough time to talk to D or visit him as much as I'd like to. And since I am working so much, I definitely don't have time for myself anymore.

S: So, you feel an extra responsibility to provide financially, but you also feel like it's taking you away from Daryl, and even, yourself.

T: Yeah… I guess so.

S: Do you think that Daryl is aware of what you're experiencing?

T: Honestly, I try not to bother him with all this. He has it hard enough in here. Plus, it's not that bad. I'm okay with working harder and being out of whack right now. It's only temporary, until we can get through this.

Sean's use of multidirected sociocultural attunement allows him to delve further into Tanya's experience, allowing her a space to voice her realities within the therapy room. Voicing this historically silent view allows her partner to develop empathy for her position within the situation. Further examining this response to the loss of her personal health balance can help Sean to see the influence of individual psychology on Tanya's outlook. Individual psychology focuses on how each person makes meaning from their experience, and how that meaning is then internalized (McDowell et al., 2023). This process of meaning making, and internalization can have a deep impact on how couples behave with one another. In this circumstance, this process has been exacerbated by the restrictive setting of incarceration on the relationship, which has caused Tanya to "power through" as opposed to feeling safe to rely on others around her. Understanding Tanya's experience puts Sean in a position to validate Tanya's process and acknowledge the latent power imbalance taking place.

Sean continues his work by discussing sociohistorical context and background. This step focuses on justice as a bridge between the past and the future (van der Meiden et al., 2020). Therapists focus on understanding the full scope of the client's connection to their family and historical experiences. Understanding these pieces can help to create a picture of the sociopolitical context of a family's legacy (McDowell et al., 2023). Further exploration of Tanya's family background indicates sociocontextual ideals of being lower class Whites, struggling with experiences of addiction and poverty across generations. From the time of her kinship placement Tanya remembers thinking low of herself and decided she did not want to be a burden to her grandmother. Sean explores how the role of gender has influenced her view. Tanya recalls hearing from her mother about the burden of being a woman and having to deal with cleaning up other people's mess. With this in mind,

Tanya felt her grandmother was already in a difficult predicament of having little money, suffering health issues in her older age, and now being tasked with raising her. This moved her to learn to fend for herself, take responsibility for her life, and remain determined to handle all issues on her own.

Understanding Tanya's experience of her childhood allows Sean to identify and acknowledge the unfairness that is currently impacting her life, as well as the presence of invisible loyalty. This involves looking across generations within Tanya's family to see how she has both received and given care in intimate relationships. Loyalty is defined as "the existential bond that connects us to our origins but may be invisible to us" (McDowell et al., 2023, p. 189). Tanya's behavior of not sharing her hardships and taking on high levels of responsibility within her relationship with Daryl are demonstrations of her intergenerational loyalty to her family. In a subsequent session, Sean is able to examine Daryl's awareness of the transactional patterns Tanya carries into the relationship:

S: Daryl, you've known Tanya for some time. Has she always been such a responsible woman?

D: Most definitely. Tanya has always held it down. I mean, I never lived with no one but my family, but living with Tanya was better than being with them. She kept the place looking tight, managed all our money, cooked all the dinners. Except for breakfast, I did that. I love this woman, she holds it down.

S: That's interesting. You know Tanya to be extremely responsible, but I wonder if you know where that comes from for Tanya?

D: I guess it comes from her grandma. That's the only person she ever really had.

S: Why don't you tell us Tanya. Where does this level of being responsible come from?

T: I think it just came from, like all the things I remember my mom saying. She was always so messed up, you know, high and stuff. And I just remember her rambling on about how women always had so much thrown at them to deal with. But I could never make sense of it. It felt like she was never dealing with anything, just getting high all the time, and dropping the ball on important stuff. Like, of course we had difficulties, we were always broke because they were always blowing their money on drugs! I wasn't going to do that with my life. Whatever comes my way, I'm going to deal with it. I'm not letting it get the best of me.

S: Hmmm. It's not right that your mom wasn't able to be there for you the way you needed. You needed her to show up and be responsible for you. But her battle with addiction kept her from that. I'm sorry that didn't happen.

T: Yeah.

S: It seems like these messages about the burden of women, having to take everything on by themselves, has been influencing your family for generations.

These patterns denote the unspoken rules, and the ledger of unfairness Tanya has brought into her relationship from previous engagement with her family, community, and larger society. The message of women having an undue burden, along with messages about poverty, and not asking for help has put Tanya in a position of taking on all of the responsibility within her relationship. Acknowledging the position of both partners as they attempt to address the concerns of their relationship, Sean uses the lens of assuming people want to give. By taking this viewpoint, Sean can leverage the couple's relational commitment to explore their desire to create a fairer balance within the relationship. It is important to recognize the societal power inequities that have taken place within both Daryl's and Tanya's life. Creating space for the couple to assess the impact of racial injustice, poverty, and gender bias. Sean's expanded focus on relational justice can help to move the couple past second-order change, as a basic change in the roles and rules of their relationship. Rather, the couple can move toward third-order change and gain a higher level of understanding regarding the impact of power, and the broader societal systems within their lives.

As they work through subsequent sessions, Sean is able to use the assumption that people want to give, to engage the clients about the current support systems in their life. Once the couple is able to value each other's experience of injustice and harm, Sean helps the couple to encourage due crediting within their family relationships. This process helps the client to give credit to others for the positive contributions they have made in their life (Hargrave & Pfritzer, 2004). A balance is created as Sean acknowledges what each client was owed by their system (love, care, safety, etc.), along with what they received. Daryl was able to acknowledge his mother doing the best she could to raise him and his sister. While Tanya was able to recognize the contribution of her grandmother for taking her in and introducing her to art as a way to channel her emotions, as she was processing the loss of her parents.

Using a socioculturally attuned contextual family therapy lens allows Sean to think about the connection of relational accountability and societal power dynamics (McDowell et al., 2023). As Daryl is currently incarcerated, his predicament may appear to force Tanya into a more responsible role. This responsibility can appear to be situated in Tanya being on the "outside". However, societal gender norms related to the role of women may influence Tanya to perform expected roles such as caretaking of the home, caring for the animals, and sole financial responsibility. Yet, as we acknowledge the societal assumptions about gender roles, we can explore ways to encourage accountability from Daryl, as he has benefited from the imbalance in the relationship:

S: It seems like Tanya has been doing a lot to make sure things continue to move as smoothly as possible since you've been here. She's managing the apartment, the dogs, working extra hours, all while trying to make sure you are okay here.

D: Yeah.

S: She's been driving the hour here, every week to engage in these therapy sessions.

D: (Looking at Tanya). Yeah, she has.

S: She's had to divert a lot of her energy, mentally, emotionally, to keep things going. And I know you can see how it's affecting her.

D: Yeah. (tears in eyes).

S: I know you love this woman, and you may feel like you can't help her from in here.

D: (Shakes head while covering face).

T: But I am wondering if you're open to brainstorming some ways you can be here for her?

Sean uses the guideline of encouraging accountability to show Daryl how he can demonstrate responsibility and accountability to others from his position as an incarcerated person. This is an important notion, as it allows Daryl to evaluate ways that he can be empowered to have an impact on his relationship, while being incarcerated. Through their generative talks, Daryl was able to understand how he was solely relying on Tanya for his needs while in prison. By assuming that people want to give to both Daryl and Tanya during this time of being separated, Sean was able to explore ways in which their familial relationships could be of value. Daryl was able to consider the role his mother and sister could play in assisting the couple. Through family talks, Daryl was able to navigate an arrangement for his little sister to feed and walk the dogs on her way home from school daily. This arrangement exemplifies his ability to gain help from his support system in a way that decreases the distress felt by his absence. Daryl was also able to speak with his mother and Tanya together to find ways to alleviate financial stress impacting him in prison. The pair was able to come up with a schedule where they traded off managing the cost of putting money on Daryl's books and where they carpooled to the facility for in-person visits. Daryl's involvement in creating these solutions helped with showing his commitment to Tanya and empowered him to demonstrate agency in managing his relationships.

Having gained support in managing the gaps left by Daryl's incarceration, Tanya was also encouraged toward accountability in her family relationships. She was able to give due credit to her grandmother for raising her and nurturing her talents as an artist. Having more energy, Tanya refocused her efforts on bringing balance and well-being to her existence. With a socioculturally attuned contextual family therapy lens, Sean was able to support Tanya in evaluating how she could be intentional about interrupting societal injustices and envisioning the impact she wanted to make within her family and local community. Tanya was becoming intentional about balancing the ledger of fairness within her family relationships. This includes acknowledging openly the positive contributions the client has made to others and that others have made to them (Goldenthal, 1996). Boszormenyi-Nagy (1987) noted that entitlement could be earned by caring for others. By attuning to others, clients are now able to approach relational interactions with empathy (McDowell et al., 2023). By recognizing the privilege she held in her life, being a White, abled-bodied, cis gendered woman, Tanya was ready to be more responsive to others, creating a pathway to constructive entitlement. Tanya now felt prepared to share her current experience with her grandmother. She found value in spending time with her grandmother at her nursing facility, where they could have conversations to encourage her learning about her family history. She also found the process of creating art with her grandmother to be one that brought her much peace. Tanya explored the idea of leading a weekly art activity for her grandmother and the other women at her facility.

Sean supported the couple as they focused forward on ways to intentionally demonstrate their commitment to one another, and their community. As the couple learns about the influence of sociopolitical realities impacting their interpersonal relationships, they can open additional space to think more deeply about how they can interrupt their experience of injustice. While Daryl and Tanya have at least two years of his sentence to weather, Sean assists the couple to envision working in partnership through this time frame. This shifts the couple from a viewpoint of helplessness to agency. McDowell et al. (2023) explained that despite the injustice they endured, family members' mutual support enabled exoneration and fresh starts, allowing them to reimagine fairness and transform their relationships through awareness of systemic oppression. This demonstrates how socioculturally attuned contextual family therapy can generate third-order change within Daryl and Tanya's current and future relationship, by creating an ethical balance.

In conclusion, this case example did not include a couple that also has children and therefore, not coparenting together. This case did not include the challenges that have been documented for incarcerated coparents. This chapter was written for incarcerated couples, things look very different post-release.

Conclusion

When supporting couples facing the challenges of incarceration, MFTs must recognize the complex systems surrounding the couple. These systems are deeply connected to each partner's unique identities, experiences, and histories. Incarceration itself acts as a significant stressor that creates strain in the couple's relationship and amplifies unresolved issues. Old wounds may resurface, including personal or generational traumas, as well as experiences of injustice. Meanwhile, unhealthy patterns of interaction may exacerbate the already difficult circumstances. In order to create change in the couple system, MFTs must be able to create a degree of safety for each member as they move through the uncertainty, isolation, and loss of incarceration. While both partners may struggle with a lack of trust in the systems around them, building trust *within* their relationship and with their clinician is essential. Trust begins with honesty. MFTs must be willing to confront the *full* reality of incarceration and its effects – not just its impact on the incarcerated individual, but also on the partners and families left behind. Recognizing these experiences fosters connection and lays the groundwork for healing for the entire family system.

References

Antle, K., Gibson, C. L., & Krohn, M. D. (2020). The mediating role of family dynamics in the relationship between paternal incarceration and child behavior problems. *Journal of Crime and Justice, 43*(1), 16–35. https://doi.org/10.1080/0735648X.2019.1619615

Arditti, J. A., Lambert-Shute, J., & Joest, K. (2003). Saturday morning at the jail: Implications of incarceration for families and children. *Family Relations, 52*(3), 195–204. https://doi.org/10.1111/j.1741-3729.2003.00195.x

Boszormenyi-Nagy, I. (1987). *Foundation of contextual therapy: Collected papers of Ivan Boszormenyi-Nagy, M.D.* Brunner/Mazel.

Bruns, A. (2019). The third shift: Multiple job holding and the incarceration of women's partners. *Social Science Research, 80*, 202–215. https://doi.org/10.1016/j.ssresearch.2018.12.024

Charles, P., Muentner, L., Jensen, S., Packard, C., Haimson, C., Eason, J., & Poehlmann-Tynan, J. (2021). Incarcerated during a pandemic: Implications of covid-19 for jailed individuals and their families. *Corrections*, 1–12. https://doi.org/10.1080/23774657.2021.2011803

Cooper, H. L., Caruso, B., Barham, T., Embry, V., Dauria, E., Clark, C. D., & Comfort, M. L. (2015). Partner incarceration and African-American women's sexual relationships and risk: A longitudinal qualitative study. *Journal of Urban Health, 92*(3), 527–547. https://doi.org/10.1007/s11524-015-9941-8

Davey-Rothwell, M. A., Villarroel, M. A., Grieb, S. D., & Latkin, C. A. (2013). Norms, attitudes, and sex behaviors among women with incarcerated main partners. *Journal of Urban Health, 90*, 1151–1165. https://doi.org/10.1007/s11524-012-9749-8

DeHart, D., Shapiro, C., & Clone, S. (2018). "The pill line is longer than the chow line": The impact of incarceration on prisoners and their families. *The Prison Journal (Philadelphia, Pa.), 98*(2), 188–212. https://doi.org/10.1177/0032885517753159

Durante, K. A., Tadros, E., Braxton, C., & Barbini, M. (2023). Supportive communication skills as a protective factor among couples experiencing incarceration. *Criminal Justice and Behavior, 50*(11), 1643–1660.https://doi.org/10.1177/00938548231195036

Dwyer Emory, A. (2022). To stay or go: Relationship dissolution and repartnering after paternal incarceration. *Family Relations, 71*(3), 1191–1210. https://doi.org/10.1111/fare.12657

Gale, L. (2022, February 18). *Biopsychosocial-spiritual assessment: An overview.* Social Work Practice and Skill: Biopsychosocial Spiritual-Assessment. https://www.ebsco.com/sites/default/files/acquiadam-assets/Social-Work-Reference-Center-Skill-Biopsychosocial-Spiritual-Assessment.pdf

Goldenthal, P. (1996). *Doing contextual therapy: An integrated model for working with individuals, couples, and families.* W.W. Norton.

Hargrave, T. D., & Pfitzer, F. (2004). *The new contextual therapy: Guiding the power of give and take* (1st ed.). Routledge. https://doi.org/10.4324/9780203501368

Kroenke, K., & Spitzer, R. L. (2002). The PHQ-9: A new depression diagnostic and severity measure. *Psychiatric Annals, 32(9)*, 509–515. https://doi.org/10.3928/0048-5713-20020901-06

McDowell, T., Knudson-Martin, C., & Bermudez, J. M. (2023). Socioculturally attuned contextual family therapy. In *Socioculturally attuned family therapy* (2nd ed., pp. 187–208). Routledge. https://doi.org/10.4324/9781003216520-9

McKay, T., Lindquist, C., Steffey, D., Feinberg, R., Landwehr, J., & Bir, A. (2018). Family life before and during incarceration. *Journal of Offender Rehabilitation, 57*(2), 96–114. https://doi.org/10.1080/10509674.2018.1441209

Pech, A., Curran, M., Speirs, K., Li, X., Barnett, M., & Paschall, K. (2020). Understanding child behavior problems in young children with previously incarcerated fathers: Parents' depressive symptoms, relationship quality, and coparenting. *Marriage & Family Review, 56*(6), 553–574. https://doi-org.libezproxy2.syr.edu/10.1080/01494929.2020.1728602

Sibley, D. S., Schmidt, A. E., & Kimmes, J. G. (2015). Applying a contextual therapy framework to treat panic disorder: A case study. *Journal of Family Psychotherapy, 26*, 299–317.

Simons, R. L., & Barr, A. B. (2014). Shifting perspectives: Cognitive changes mediate the impact of romantic relationships on desistance from crime. *Justice Quarterly, 31*(5), 793–821. https://doi.org/10.1080/07418825.2012.704388

Skardhamar, T., Savolainen, J., Aase, K. N., & Lyngstad, T. H. (2015). Does marriage reduce crime? *Crime & Justice (Chicago, Ill), 44*(1), 385–446. https://doi.org/10.1086/681557

Skipper, A. D., Bates, D. S., Blizard, Z. D., & Moye, R. G. (2020). Charged with instability: Are paternal arrests and criminal charges enough to shake the marital stability of American couples? *Journal of Family Issues, 41*(12), 2423–2447. https://doi.org/10.1177/0192513X20942813

Spanier, G. B. (1976). Measuring dyadic adjustment: New scales for assessing the quality of marriage and similar dyads. *Journal of Marriage and the Family, 38*(1), 15–28. https://doi.org/10.2307/350547

Spitzer, R. L., Kroenke, K., Williams, J. B., & Löwe, B. (2006). A brief measure for assessing generalized anxiety disorder: the GAD-7. *Archives of Internal Medicine, 166*(10), 1092–1097. https://doi.org/10.1001/archinte.166.10.1092

Sumra, M. K., & Schillaci, M. A. (2015). Stress and the multiple-role woman: Taking a closer look at the "superwoman". *PLoS ONE*, 10(3), Article e0120952. https://doi.org/10.1371/journal.pone.0120952

Tadros, E., & Ansell, A. (2022). Romantic attachment, childhood stability, depression, and PTSD in couples with an incarcerated partner. *Journal of Forensic Sciences, 67*(2), 619–629. https://doi.org/10.1111/1556-4029.14976

Tadros, E., Durante, K. A., McKay, T., Barbini, M., Hollie, B., Shepardson, R. L., & Polaha, J. (2022a). Mental health, perceived consensus of coparenting, and physical health among incarcerated fathers and their nonincarcerated, romantic partners. *Families Systems & Health, 40*(2), 210–224. https://doi.org/10.1037/fsh0000671

Tadros, E., Durante, K. A., McKay, T., & Hollie, B. (2022b). Coparenting from prison: An examination of incarcerated fathers' consensus of coparenting. *The American Journal of Family Therapy, 50*(3), 314–332. https://doi.org/10.1080/01926187.2021.1913669

Tadros, E., & Finney, N. (2018). Structural family therapy with incarcerated families. *The Family Journal, 26*(2), 253–261.

Tadros, E., Presley, S., & Gomez, E. (2022c). "Not for the Weak": The lived experience of women in romantic relationships with incarcerated individuals. *Crime and Delinquency, 68*(12), 2274–2297. https://doi.org/10.1177/00111287221077657

Tadros, E., Presley, S., & Gomez, E. (2023). Incarcerated loved ones: Building a community to support and advocate on facebook. *International Journal of Environmental Research and Public Health, 20*(5), 4002-. https://doi.org/10.3390/ijerph20054002

Tadros, E., & Vlach, A. (2023). Conflictual couples: The impact of dyadic adjustment and depressive symptoms on conflict in incarcerated couples. *Journal of Family Trauma, Child Custody & Child Development (Print), 20*(2), 239–257. https://doi.org/10.1080/26904586.2022.2041525

Turney, K. (2015). Hopelessly devoted? Relationship quality during and after incarceration. *Journal of Marriage and Family, 77*(2), 480–495.

Turney, K., & Wildeman, C. (2013). Redefining relationships: Explaining the countervailing consequences of paternal incarceration for parenting. *American Sociological Review, 78*(6), 949–979. https://doi.org/10.1177/0003122413505589

van der Meiden, J., Verduijn, K., Noordegraaf, M. and van Ewijk, H. (2020), Strengthening Connectedness in Close Relationships: A Model for Applying Contextual Therapy. *Family Process*, 59: 346–360. https://doi.org/10.1111/famp.12425

Wallace, D., Larson, M., Somers, L., Padilla, K. E., & Mays, R. (2020). Recidivism and relationships: Examining the role of relationships, transitions, and relationship quality in reincarceration. *Journal of Developmental and Life-Course Criminology, 6*, 321–352. https://doi.org/10.1007/s40865-020-00144-6

Wildeman, C., Lee, H., & Comfort, M. (2013). A new vulnerable population? The health of female partners of men recently released from prison. *Women's Health Issues, 23*(6), e335–e340. https://doi.org/10.1016/j.whi.2013.07.006

Yeboaa, P. A., Mbamba, C. R., & Ndemole, I. K. (2022). "Everything Has Turned Against Us": Experiences of left-behind spouses of incarcerated persons. *Journal of Social Service Research, 48*(3), 345–352. https://doi.org/10.1080/01488376.2022.2042456

Chapter 5

Relational Interventions within Carceral Settings

Brooke M. Tindall and Kevin T. Long

As explored throughout this book, incarceration can have catastrophic consequences for families, as the removal of someone from a home affects relationships, finances, mental health, and the overall stability of a household. The majority of incarcerated people were already surviving marginalization and societal disadvantage prior to their arrest, as the United States's justice system disproportionately targets oppressed groups navigating necropolitical spaces (Elderbroom et al., 2018; McKay et al., 2018a). The removal of a close family member from society is financially and structurally devastating as families are often burdened with the loss of housing, health insurance, and financial stability following the loss of an income earner (Comfort et al., 2016; Geller et al., 2009). When disadvantaged people are removed from disadvantaged households, the family left behind is often plunged into even worse desperation, which the country tactfully reframes as depravity so they can perpetuate a cyclical pattern of disadvantage, crime, and punishment through generations of oppressed groups.

Support Systems and Recidivism

The family, whether biological or found, is the first ring of support for any person in human society (Silk & Goldman, 2013). They have the most potential to be the first line of defense against suffering due to their shared history, knowledge, and proximity to the person and problem. The population that faces the most societal disadvantage and is in the most need of support is the most prone to losing their family to the carceral system. The carceral system's degradation of the family is emotionally devastating for everyone affected and withers away at the resilience of these struggling populations (McKay et al., 2016).

The current American carceral system is not designed to support incarcerated people and their families in maintaining or improving connections, so families often struggle to maintain bonds during a family member's incarceration. This lack of opportunity for connection is especially counterproductive for those who were victims, participants, or perpetrators of

DOI: 10.4324/9781003542940-5

dysfunctional family dynamics prior to their arrest. Their reality may be marked by leaving a broken family, spending years disconnected and alienated with very few opportunities to repair their relationships, and returning home to estranged loved ones harboring resentment for their unsettled disputes and feelings of abandonment. Returning to a tense family at risk of crisis is a pipeline for engaging in harmful stress-induced behaviors such as drug use that could lead to reentry failure (Liu & Visher, 2021). Family and relationship therapists believe that providing individuals with a strong support system, particularly through a stable family, is often the most effective way to prevent recidivism.

The importance of prioritizing the well-being of family systems must not be understated. For many decades, researchers have hyper-focused on advocating for and increasing structural support for released people, and such efforts have been effective. It is easier for released individuals to find housing and employment than in the past, as many organizations have banned together to create structural support systems. However, individuals reentering society report that even with solid structural support from community resources, they still feel unsupported (Denney et al., 2014). Community aid is not enough. A system or organization is not capable of offering the same personal relationship that individual human beings can offer. Thus, those reentering society long for support from social circles, desperate for more social connectedness, especially with their families.

Those who are able to connect with their families and utilize their family's resources, such as job connections, transportation, and housing, have an easier time reintegrating into society due to greater stability and social connectivity. Social connections are so valuable as friends and family enforce accountability and instill released loved ones with a sense of purpose that can motivate them to commit to rehabilitation and successful reentry (Denney et al., 2014). Empirical research corroborates that the positive outcomes of strong family bonds that allow for structural and social support ultimately result in lower recidivism rates (Bales & Mears, 2008; Datchi & Sexton, 2013; Vera Institute of Justice, 2011). This highlights the importance of incarcerated people staying connected to their families during incarceration so that they may rely on their loved ones' hearts and homes following release (Denney et al., 2014; Folk et al., 2019).

Lower recidivism has benefits beyond the incarcerated person's potential and well-being. Healthy relationships are mutual. The more stable and rehabilitated an individual is post-release, the less their family will be subjected to further maladaptive behavior and retraumatizing events. In addition to preventing negative experiences, therapy allows people to learn to contribute to their family's ring of support and participate in mutually beneficial relationships.

Positive social integration enhances far more than just the well-being of incarcerated individuals and their families. Family therapy in prisons could yield broader societal benefits by helping families transform from a source of community strain into a source of community resilience. The personal growth of incarcerated people and their families can prevent generational cycles of disadvantage, protect public safety, reduce the economic toll of crime, and alleviate burden on correctional facilities and social services. An investment in family therapy is an investment in every layer of the fabric of society: individual, family, community, and institution.

Correctional Facilities and Family Connection

Barriers to Communication

While cartoonish, many people often think of the stereotypical "You get one phone call!" line shouted by a police officer when someone has just been arrested. While this is usually delivered as a joke for laughs on television, in reality, this moment marks the beginning of a long period of excessively limited and complicated opportunities for connection. Throughout the literature, incarcerated people repeatedly report on the extent of barriers to connection and the strain they put on relationships (Durante et al., 2024; Dutcher & Barnes-Ceeney, 2021; Naser & Visher, 2006; Rubenstein et al., 2021; Turney et al., 2023).

Phone calls are not only limited, they are also expensive. Video calls can be expensive and vary across states and facilities. To talk to someone in the Westmoreland County Prison in Pennsylvania, it would cost $15 per 25 minutes. Simple phone calls range from being free to $3.15 per 15 minutes, depending on state legislature (Wagner & Bertram, 2022). Three dollars may not seem like much to the average American, but imagine a single mother of three children trying to ensure everyone gets 15 minutes to talk to their incarcerated family member a week. By the end of the month, they would have spent $50 dollars on calls. Such a price on simple communication can force loved ones to abbreviate their calls, cutting short what may be the only method through which they connect. There is a consequence to treating phone calls like a luxury and locking them behind a paywall when most of the population trying to use the service is impoverished. There is hope on the horizon for the government to regulate the cost of these calls, with recent legislation passed under the Biden Administration (Martha Wright-Reed Just and Reasonable Communications Act of 2022, 2022). Even so, the barriers still exist so long as there is a paywall.

Perhaps the ease or affordability of making a call would seem less problematic if in-person visitations were not nearly impossible. The American carceral system's policies are blatantly isolationist, with the Justice system setting a precedent that placing someone in a federal facility up to 500 miles (805 km) away or a state facility up to 100 miles (161 km) away from their community is standard procedure (U.S. Department of Justice, 2019). For context, the amount of time one would have to drive to reach such facilities for visitation is around 8.5 hours and 2 hours, respectively. Such a distance with the cost of travel, loss of income, and time out of school may not be worth the reward of a time-limited visitation. Even in a state as liberal as New York, incarcerated people are granted a maximum of only two visitations a week, so there is a level of coordination necessary to ensure there will be a visit at the end of a long road trip (The Legal Aid Society, 2024).

Conjugal visits may seem more worth the effort, but they are only offered in four states. Being able to consider whether the trek is worth it is a privilege, with 34% of participants in one study reporting they could not visit their family members regardless of cost or time because they did not even have transportation (Naser & Visher, 2006). The barrier of distance possibly has the greatest effect on the incarcerated individuals' isolation as distance is associated with fewer in-person visitations (Clark & Duwe, 2017; Cochran et al., 2016).

All of these barriers to connection have financial implications with the cost of calls, travel, and sending packages or letters, needing to be contextualized as potentially unreasonable for a financially struggling family with one less pillar of financial support. These barriers appear even more pronounced when the average length of prison sentences in America is considered. In federal prisons, the average stay is 147 months or 12.3 years, which is an awfully long time to be so incredibly disconnected from someone (United States Sentencing Commission, 2021).

A large reason why access to family members is so restricted is the need for prisons to minimize risk around incarcerated people having outside contacts whom they can use to exchange information related to gang relations, or illegal operations. Visitations also create opportunities for visitors to deliver contraband to incarcerated people. Such risks lead facilities to weigh the benefits of allowing incarcerated people to contact others with the reality of staffing and security limitations (Fulcher, 2013). These facilities have decided that prison safety is their priority. However, their approach to minimizing risk is ineffective and actually creates more risk as incarcerated people's mental health and familial stability crumble as a consequence of systemic neglect and alienation.

Prison Systems Sponsoring Connections

Considering the importance of maintaining and repairing family bonds, prison systems that encourage connection by sponsoring quality family time boast the lowest recidivism rates for their ex-convicts. Norway is a prime example, as its prison system in the 1990s closely resembled the USA's current system, with a focus on punishment and removal from society. In the 1990s, Norway's recidivism rate was 70% within two years of release, comparable to the USA's current rate of 68% within three years of release (Butler & Taylor, 2022). Over the last 30 years, Norway has completely reformed its prison system. Among the most relevant changes to family dynamics was the movement away from large, centralized prisons to small community-based prisons. Despite having a relatively small population, the country has 57 prisons. The prisons are relatively tiny, with some having less than 20 cells. Norway's prison system is accessible and welcoming to families as those who are detained are sent to local facilities close to their communities. Family visitation is encouraged up to three times a week and some of the prisons allow for conjugal visitations. Norway also greatly reduced the length of its prison sentences with 90% of sentences being less than a year long (First Step Alliance, 2022). These changes are vital for family connectedness, as they allow incarcerated people to avoid alienation and disconnectedness from their families.

To replicate Norway's prison system, the USA would have to reform and restructure its entire correctional system, including policies, building locations, and corporate contracts, which is highly unlikely to occur within the foreseeable future. Thus, our challenge is to channel Norway's emphasis on family connection within the USA's barrier-riddled isolationist prison system. Relationship and family therapists have been proposing, funding, and researching therapeutic services to help incarcerated Americans maintain and strengthen connections with their families within the current system.

Family Therapy

Even if incarcerated individuals had more access to their families, does mere connection suffice to maintain bonds? The unique challenges faced by incarcerated individuals and their families before, during, and after incarceration often strain relationships beyond what visitation or phone calls can address. Imprisonment can create complex emotional dynamics affected by guilt, anger, longing, and a sense of abandonment that require deep, vulnerable, and honest conversations to address. Expensive, time-restrictive, and public communication is not conducive to allowing space for the kinds of conversations necessary for relational repair. People who are incarcerated also often come from families with maladaptive communication patterns and may lack communication skills that allow them to listen without becoming defensive and frustrated. The combination of internal, environmental, and relational barriers to repair is overwhelming as fruitless bids for connection and conversations that end in conflict become undeniably discouraging. The communication they currently have with their families is often not sufficient enough to create healthy and mutually beneficial support systems.

It is evident that having professional guidance to navigate attempts at repair would benefit incarcerated people and their families (Datchi et al., 2016). As MFTs, we aim to help families struggling with incarceration to create opportunities to repair and strengthen their relationships through relational therapeutic services. Relationship and family therapy is a systemic psychotherapy that focuses treatment on the relationships between people rather than on the individual people within a relational system. The primary goal of systemic therapies is to understand the dynamics, patterns, and communication styles within a system and facilitate positive change by providing systems with alternative ways of interacting. This approach recognizes that imprisonment affects the whole family, and by addressing relational issues, the overall health and strength of the family unit can improve.

Family therapy could provide incarcerated people and their loved ones with the tools to:

1 Strengthen and maintain bonds despite physical separation: Professional guidance can help families nurture their relationships even when they are physically separated due to incarceration. Family therapists can introduce strategies and interventions to cultivate a sense of presence in each other's lives through meaningful interactions, rituals, and traditions that create a sense of togetherness and continuity. This can make space for moments of connection that give family members something to look forward to before their interactions and something to remember fondly following their interactions. Having shared moments helps individuals feel as though they are part of each other's lives. It gives them memories they can reflect on when they are apart and reminisce over when they are together, contributing to feelings of companionship, connectedness, and oneness.
2 Build relational awareness: Family therapists can offer a third-party perspective that helps incarcerated individuals and their families identify how societal issues, relational patterns, and personal dynamics interconnect, which promotes a deeper understanding of how each member's actions affect the whole family unit. They can gain insights into how their behaviors and interactions may unintentionally contribute to each other's struggles. By bringing these patterns to light, therapists enable families to see the broader context of the problems, which are often obscured by stress or limited perspective. Insight into their relationship dynamics is crucial for developing effective strategies to break negative cycles that perpetuate their presenting problem(s) and foster healthier relationships.
3 Develop healthier ways of interacting: Family therapy can assist individuals in developing more productive communication strategies, including active listening, communicating emotion, setting boundaries, expressing empathy, and sharing supportive messages. Therapists can also alter ways

of interacting that are destructive to bonds, such as aggression, criticism, and defense mechanisms that prevent meaningful and fulfilling interactions. In time, families could learn to resolve conflicts without resorting to negative behaviors. By learning and practicing healthier communication skills, families can transform their interactions from sources of conflict into opportunities for connection and understanding.

4 Develop coping strategies for dealing with the stress of separation: Both incarcerated people and their families endure significant emotional strain due to separation. Therapy can equip them with techniques to manage this stress effectively. This might include stress-reduction practices, building emotional resilience, and creating broader support networks outside the family unit, ensuring that they have additional sources of emotional support and practical assistance. By developing coping strategies, families can better manage the challenges of separation, reducing the risk of emotional burnout and strengthening their ability to support themselves and each other.
5 Address and resolve conflicts that arise due to incarceration: The stress of incarceration often leads to misunderstandings and conflicts. Family therapy offers a structured environment to address these issues constructively. Therapists provide a neutral space where family members can express their concerns and feelings in productive ways, as therapists encourage healthier dialogue and minimize avoidance, blame, or deflection. By having a mediator, families are able to have deeper, more honest conversations than they would normally be able to achieve on their own. Family therapy allows families to navigate difficult conversations, mediate disputes, and develop healthier ways of confronting one another which ultimately allows them to spend less time arguing and more time supporting each other.
6 Prepare for eventual reintegration into family life post-release: Family therapy can help families prepare for challenging transitions by setting realistic expectations, planning for changes in family dynamics, and developing a supportive environment that facilitates released individuals' adjustment to life outside of prison. Therapists can guide families in discussing and planning for the practical and emotional aspects of reintegration, such as finding employment, re-establishing roles of family hierarchy, rebuilding trust, and taking steps to ensure the incarcerated person does not repeat the same mistakes that led to their incarceration. By addressing potential challenges and developing strategies to manage them, therapy helps families create a supportive and structured environment that promotes the successful reintegration of the formerly incarcerated individual into family and community life.

Unfortunately, most American jails and prisons barely offer individual therapy, much less relational therapy. Furthermore, any therapy that *is* offered is of a lower quality due to the privatization of institutions and cost of services

(Daniel, 2007). As a result, this crucial resource is unavailable to the vast majority of people living behind bars, leaving their connections vulnerable to the corrosive effects of stress, separation, alienation, stigma, and resentment. Without professional support, these emotional challenges can erode family bonds, leading to a breakdown in relationships that could otherwise serve as a source of stability and resiliency.

Current Therapeutic Approaches to Incarcerated People and Their Families

Researchers have implemented programs sponsoring relational therapy in carceral facilities to understand the effectiveness of such programs in improving familial bonds and creating positive life outcomes for released people. Such programs typically adhere to the risk-need-responsivity (RNR) principle, tailoring care based on families' specific needs and risks to ensure families with greater needs receive more comprehensive support (Andrews & Bonta, 2010). However, the factors prisons use to judge whether someone receives support must be flawed, as there are many populations not receiving care adequate enough to prevent future detainments. The following section explores the existing therapeutic interventions (or lack of interventions) for juveniles, adults, romantic partners, and parents. We provide justifications for the need for specific interventions through case examples and empirical literature. This program review concludes with a discussion of best practices and considerations for further implementation of relational therapy in prison settings.

Juveniles and Their Families

Jazon's Story

Jazon (15M) is currently being held in a detention center and has been meeting with a counselor to assess what resources would be best for supporting him. Jazon's has described his parents as neglectful. When he was a toddler, they would leave him home alone with his older brother while they were at work. His older brother, who was also a young child, would terrorize him for hours in their parents' absence. Jazon's mother and father are married, hardworking, emotionally distant, and very critical of their children. They often referred to Jazon as a financial burden and led him to feel like an inconvenience. They would spank him for minor mistakes and often during misunderstandings. Jazon did not feel loved, wanted, understood, or safe. He critically lacked attention and connection at home. School did not provide him with the support he was lacking, as his attention-seeking behaviors were often punished in the school environment and he was treated as a barrier to his classmates learning.

The consequences of Jazon lacking a supportive and caring environment were depressive, anxious, and apathetic symptomatology. He frequently ran away from home and skipped school. He desperately searched for belonging and understanding in his community and utilized drugs to cope with the psychological consequences of his upbringing. He built a support system composed of other misunderstood teens, unhoused youth, and older folks that would occasionally provide shelter, drugs, and protection. He also began using marijuana and experimenting with illicit substances.

His friends and he began stealing cars and posting videos of their thefts online. This behavior went without consequence until they were driving under the influence in a stolen car and swerved into a business after accidentally crashing into a young couple who were walking their dog in the night. Jazon was driving the car at the time of the incident and fell unconscious, though he sustained no physical injuries from the accident.

When asked what he would like his life to look like, Jazon responded:

> I don't know. Honestly this ain't too bad. Ain't no one ever cared about me outside of here. The people who know me and got my back are either on the streets or they are in here. If you want me to go back to my parents you're trippin. They don't want me. They never did.

Jazon's friends, drug usage, and criminal activities appear to all stem from his experience of rejection in his family and school. Concerned for Jazon's lack of a stable and supportive system, the counselor refers him for a high-intensity early intervention program with a focus on healing his relationship with his family system and reengaging in school with better academic and social support.

Many kids who get involved in the criminal justice system have stories with similar themes to Jazon's. Their stories are marked by untreated trauma as well as abuse, rejection, and neglect from their attachment figures (Basto-Pereira et al., 2022). Such experiences often lead them to cope in maladaptive ways, attach themselves to negative role models and sometimes become apathetic.

By intervening at the crucial developmental state of adolescence, programs can equip youth and their families with the skills, knowledge, and support systems necessary for them to better navigate their own lives and proactively integrate into society. Most programs aiming to support incarcerated populations target adolescents primarily because youth who become involved with the justice system at a young age are likely to remain entangled with the legal system into adulthood without intervention (Loeber et al., 2013). Initiatives for youth and their families operate on the principle that early intervention can divert them from a path of continued criminal engagement and redirect them toward more positive outcomes. Disrupting adolescents' potential trajectory toward reoffending as adults is vital for supporting positive life outcomes, as adults are far more harshly punished by the justice system than adolescents.

Early intervention is also believed to be more cost-effective than later interventions, as investments in youth can prevent the overall burden on the criminal justice system and associated social services by reducing or eliminating future offenses. Because the overall goal of such programs is to avoid rearrest, the intensity of early interventions varies in frequency, length, content, and care team composition depending on how much support a youth is assessed to need in order to promote better life outcomes. The intensity of interventions increases with the likelihood of a youth's rearrest, with the most intense services targeting youth with co-occurring disorders and serious legal convictions and the least intense services targeting at-risk youth. The interventions are outlined below in order of intensity, beginning with the most intense and comprehensive intervention.

Family Integrative Transition Therapy

Intense comprehensive interventions are available for youth who commit serious offenses or have complex psychological and relational dynamics. Family Integrative Transition Therapy (FIT) is the most intense of all of the therapies and is only offered to youth in juvenile rehabilitation facilities who meet specific criteria such as having co-occurring disorders. The therapy is inspired by Multisystemic Therapy (MST), Motivational Enhancement Therapy, Relapse Prevention, and Dialectical Behavior Therapy (Aos, 2004). FIT is delivered through a team of four therapists. All teams have a child mental health specialist and a chemical dependency specialist. There are benefits to having such a team, such as being able to provide highly specialized and targeted services. The therapists engage the client's family, peers, neighborhood, and school system to help foster an environment conducive to positive behavioral and functional changes. On average, FIT lasts longer than the other therapies. It starts two months prior to release and continues four to six months post-release for a total duration of six to eight months. Those who participate in FIT have shown a decrease in recidivism across degrees of crime, with youths showing 6% decrease in chance to commit misdemeanors, 14% decrease in felonies, and 3% decrease in violent felonies.

Multisystemic Therapy

MST approaches are less intense and expensive, having just one therapist act as an individual therapist, family therapist, and social worker (Henggeler et al., 1992; Henggeler & Schaeffer, 2016). Therapists connect with clients' schools, peers, families, and any other systems that clients request the therapist connect with. The approach is highly informed by systems perspectives as therapists target interactions within family, peer, and school systems. Clinicians seek to transform parent-child relationships by improving emotional bonds and teaching guardians effective parenting and discipline methods. Therapists work with peer groups to improve adolescents' social competency and reduce the use of aggression with peers. Therapists also collaborate with adolescents' schools to help improve academic performance. MST has been effective in improving family cohesion and reducing arrests, offenses, and time incarcerated. Clients have also reported using less aggression with their peers following the intervention. MST is impressively consistent in effectiveness across populations, being equally effective with youth of varying genders and ethnicities.

Multidimensional Family Therapy

Multidimensional family therapy (MDFT) is also an intensive and involved therapy where one therapist fulfills multiple roles and involves themselves in many facets of their clients lives to unify sources of support. MDFT has therapists follow adolescents from the detention center to the months following their release, with ten hours a month of treatment for three or more months (Liddle, 2014; Simons et al., 2017). In addition to therapy, the clinician attends court hearings, school hearings, and communicates with justice personnel to coordinate care. MDFT has a risk minimization component that utilizes group therapies and prevention education modules that expose adolescents to content related to HIV prevention, safe sex, and substance use. MDFT targets individual mental health, family dynamics, and juvenile education. Youth who received MDFT were more satisfied with their treatment than those in control conditions. It is notable that retention rates for control conditions following detention were only 13% compared to 87% for those who participated in MDFT treatment. The intervention was effective in inspiring decreased substance use, fewer instances of unprotected sex, and decreased delinquency.

Functional Family Therapy

Functional family therapy (FFT) is less comprehensive than FFT, MST, and MDFT, making it more applicable to youth with variable risk levels and affordable enough to offer to lower-risk adolescents. FFT has been used as a prevention therapy for at-risk youth, an intervention for incarcerated youth, and as an intervention for youth on probation (Sexton & Alexander, 2000). It is usually available for juveniles on probation and typically lasts two to six months, depending on the needs of the youth. FFT targets interpersonal relationships with parents and peers, maladaptive cognitions, and negative emotions (Datchi & Sexton, 2013; Sexton & Alexander, 2000; Sexton & Turner, 2010). The intervention is supported by over 40 years of research that has established it as a brief and inexpensive method for reducing recidivism and helping juveniles improve their behavior and mental health (Hartnett et al., 2017; Sexton & Alexander, 2000). When therapists strictly adhere to the treatment model, clients have less emotional and behavioral problems. They also commit less risk behaviors, misdemeanors, violent crimes, and felonies than control groups. It is notable that the effectiveness of FFT may vary across race, gender, and age, suggesting there is room for the intervention to become more mindful and attuned to intersectionality (Celinska et al., 2013).

Brief Strategic Family Therapy

Brief Strategic Family Therapy (BSFT) is for lower risk adolescents and focuses less on mental health and more on how guardians treat their child and the strategies they use to operate their household. BSFT is problem-focused, and aims to alter the behavior of parents, believing that parents' behavior will either promote or punish the adolescent's behavior (Szapocznik et al., 2012; Szapocznik & Williams, 2000). BSFT typically lasts 8–24 sessions, or about two to six months. The advantages of BSFT are that it is inexpensive and easy to implement as it requires less time and resources than most other interventions, making it ideal for youth with less extreme risk factors. BSFT is effective across various races in improving family functioning. It often yields better results than other child and adolescent therapies.

Multiple Family Group Intervention

Perhaps the least individualized and intense of all the therapies is the Multiple Family Group Intervention (MFGI). Group therapy sessions bring multiple families together to participate in joint therapy and support activities. MFGI is often a more practical way to involve families in the rehabilitation process as therapies that grant families personalized and direct attention can be prohibitively expensive and time-consuming, making them challenging to implement in government-funded prison systems with lower risk adolescents. An example of an MFGI is Keiley's (2007) group targeting attachment and affect regulation with the goal of reducing recidivism and the externalizing of behavior. The group ran for eight sessions and despite being so short was seemingly effective with participants boasting a recidivism rate of 44%, which is lower than typical national averages of 65–85%. For adolescents and their families, the benefit of group therapy is a sense of normalization, community, understanding, and joint accountability.

While beneficial, convenient, brief, and cost-effective there are drawbacks to such generalized interventions. In a group setting, it can be challenging to address the specific needs and unique dynamics of each family. The presence of multiple families means that the focus and attention of the facilitators are divided, potentially limiting the depth of intervention that any one family receives. Overall, group therapy is appealing to institutions aiming to minimize their investments in their youth and most appropriate for families who need minimal support.

In summary, programs that target juveniles seek to prevent them from repeating arrestable offenses and distance them from risky behaviors such as substance use, unsafe sex, and aggressive peer relationships. They also seek to improve familial relationships, keep parents close during incarceration, and improve the effectiveness of guardians' parenting approaches. Ensuring the safety and continued development of young people is a critical component of fighting the negative effects of the carceral system and can work to prevent a cycle of re-offense.

Adults and Their Families

After adolescence, benefactors stop funneling resources toward incarcerated people, and they are essentially given up on by the justice system and mental health community. Age is the determining factor in whether or not an individual is eligible for interventions. One major reason programs for adolescents are so successful is due to the family focus which is naturally taken with younger people, this ensures that all members of a family unit are heard and supported through whatever hardship they may be facing. Though once someone is considered an adult, most interventions shift to an individual focus rather than a family focus, which can fall short of the needs of both the individual and their family as they begin to navigate through new hardships (Sexton, 2016). Most of the interventions described below were implemented by therapists as a case study, as there are very few established and available intervention programs for adults and families impacted by the carceral system.

Multidimensional Family Therapy

One of the most effective programs for this population is actually a program for juveniles that Liddle et al. (2024) modified for young adults involved in drug courts. The multidimensional approach is advantageous for young adults reentering their communities because the therapists utilize family systems and community resources to cultivate social and structural support. For four to six months, MDFT therapists work with young adults and their families to foster relational healing and bonding while simultaneously connecting individuals to systems for case management, education, job training, and employment. This intervention is impressively effective with low drop-out and recidivism rates, decreased substance use, decreased legal risk, and improved vocational functioning.

Solution-Focused Network Therapy

Solution-Focused Network Therapy (SFNT) is unlike most other interventions in that it enables incarcerated individuals to choose what members of their social support system they want involved in their relational therapy (Lindforss & Magnusson, 1997). The therapy takes place during incarceration over two to ten months, depending on the needs of the person and their system. SFNT is future-oriented, prompting the incarcerated person and their network to develop solutions for the issues surrounding risk factors that will arise upon release, so that the network can have a plan around preventing recidivism. The therapy is effective in reducing recidivism, with the participants receiving SFNT having lower recidivism rates than the control group at the 12-month (53% vs 76%) and 16-month follow-up (60% vs 86%).

Structural Family Therapy

Structural Family Therapy (SFT) aims to examine the structure of family units in order to assess the sustainability or appropriateness of family dynamics, boundaries, roles, and hierarchies. As members of the family are forced to adapt to the changes caused by incarceration, the structure of their families massively shifts. Therapists assist clients in adapting to new structures so they can experience better family cohesion and functioning. Within SFT, this consists of helping the individual family members understand the dysfunction that is occurring in their family unit, as well as how their unique role may play into perpetuating or combating said dysfunction (Tadros et al., 2024). This can range anywhere from a parent understanding their parenting style and role in the life of their children to a child understanding the role their parent or guardian plays in a family unit as a caregiver. Considering the importance of being familiar with the dynamics and structure of the family in SFT, there is no defined duration of care as it can take weeks, months, or years for therapists to identify the dynamics of families and effectively alter them. SFT has been delivered in a carceral setting through a case study, and though the intervention does not usually have a time restraint, the facility in which the study took place restricted the intervention to six weeks, possibly limiting the potential effectiveness of the intervention (Tadros & Finney, 2018, 2019). Additionally, findings suggest that culturally informed care practices are of the utmost importance when utilizing SFT with incarcerated or formerly incarcerated individuals (Tadros et al., 2024).

Multicultural Family Therapy

Because most programs are designed for large-scale implementation, they often have a standardized approach that feels rushed and impersonal. There are a few therapies that have been delivered to incarcerated adults on a case study level, where clinicians were able to emphasize overall family well-being and take a highly tailored, individualized approach to their therapy and client. One such intervention is multicultural family therapy (Tadros et al., 2019; Tadros & Owens, 2021). It is a social justice-oriented, socioculturally attuned therapy that emphasizes how the identities of individuals can affect not only their experience of the world but also their experiences in their relationships. The justification for using such a specific intervention is that they are particularly applicable to the incarcerated population who disproportionately hold identities or are related to others with identities that are related to marginalized cultures, ethnicities, and races that impact them and their families' lived experience. This impact is especially relevant to the incarcerated population as America struggles with issues concerning police brutality and unequal treatment across all races and backgrounds. There are likely many people who have specific traumas and triggers that can be related directly to social injustice within America's ironically named justice system.

Medical Family Therapy

Another intervention delivered on a case study level is Medical Family Therapy (MedFT) (Tadros & Finney, 2019). Notably in Tadros and Finney's MedFT intervention they implemented elements of SFT as well. MedFT advocates for the application of highly individualized interventions that address and center clients' families' specific needs according to an integrated biological, psychological, and social model. MedFT therapists analyze how biological components impact other dimensions of their lives as illness often contributes to interconnected social, financial, and psychological stress. Illness can have profound impacts on families and individuals and for some, may be contributing to the problems that led to their incarceration.

MedFT emphasizes informed care that infuses disability advocacy, social justice, and therapeutic resources into an empowering and transformative intervention. The overarching goals in MedFT are to assist families in navigating the healthcare system, becoming a more effective team for facing the challenges of illness and illness treatment, creating and maintaining lifestyle changes, and healing relationships that have frayed as a result of illness, disability, and the healthcare system.

MedFT Case Example

Deborah (66F) lives with multiple sclerosis and type 1 diabetes. She relied heavily on her grandson, Jordan (21M), to assist with everyday tasks as well as monitoring her dietary needs brought on by diabetes. To support him and his grandmother, Jordan began obtaining funds through illegal means, which led to his detainment. Deborah now lives with her older sister, Janet (70F), who was already struggling prior to her sister moving in with her and does not have the energy, transportation, or money to support them. Jordan feels a great sense of guilt for not being able to support his grandmother. Deborah feels helpless, abandoned, and disappointed in Jordan. She is unable to call him without her sister's financial and physical help. Jordan tries calling Janet, but she is resentful of Jordan for many reasons. The last time Jordan was incarcerated, Janet sent him money to make calls, and she paid off his bond so he could be home while awaiting sentencing. After he was released, he never thanked her or visited her to show appreciation for the support she provided him. Janet is annoyed by Jordan being arrested for a second time and leaving Deborah in her care, and she feels entirely uninvested in his well-being. She does not wish to answer his calls or support him during his second arrest.

Sara is a licensed marriage and family therapist specializing in MedFT. Sara's goal is to provide Jordan, Janet, and Deborah with emotional support, connect them with medical resources, and help them reorganize roles and responsibilities as they navigate and adjust to life without Jordan's caretaking. To accomplish her goal of providing medical support, Sara connects Janet and Deborah to resources for help accessing affordable medicine and acquiring in-home aids that are covered by their insurance. These resources alleviate some responsibility for Janet, reduce Jordan's concern for Deborah while he's incarcerated, and could prevent him from having to commit crimes of survival following his incarceration. He can rest knowing his grandmother has other support resources.

To emotionally and systemically support the family, Sara works to repair the relationship between Jordan and Janet and bring attention to how Jordan can reciprocate the love Janet provided during his last incarceration. Sara also guides Deborah and Jordan discussing how disability has impacted their lives, what being there for each other means to each of them, and what it is like to live without each other. In doing so, Sara helps everyone process their feelings, ensures old conflicts are resolved, and creates a more welcoming environment for Jordan post-release. As the family begins utilizing medical resources and reconnecting with one other, the distribution of responsibility becomes more manageable for Janet. Sara emphasizes that Jordan and Janet do not have to be alone in caring for Deborah. They can work together to support her and perhaps also grow to support each other as well.

Romantic Partners

Overall, there are not many therapy programs designed specifically for partners affected by the carceral system. There are education programs that aim to assist couples in developing relationship skills during and following imprisonment (Goodey et al., 2019; Negash et al., 2022a). Though systemic and supportive of healthier relationships, educational interventions are not long-term or therapeutic. They also tend to be limited in scope as they are typically heteronormative and designed for monogamous couples. Thus, those seeking therapeutic relational support for their partnership have few options.

There is a need for romantic partners to have access to treatment options. Such programs would greatly benefit partners, who are impacted by the stress of incarceration both during and following release. Partners left behind are burdened with twice as many responsibilities. The emotional, financial, and structural impact of a partners' incarceration often plunge people into a depression and force them to rearrange their priorities. Perhaps this is why women are more likely to drop out of school and engage in more drug use and alcohol consumption during a male partner's incarceration (Wildeman et. al., 2013). These sacrifices are not only detrimental to the quality of these women's lives but also their partners who return home to concerns about their partner's achievements, mental health, and substance use, none of which are conducive to a smooth reentry. Because the period following a partner's prison sentence is acutely stressful, the potential for heightened physical violence between partners increases (McKay et al., 2018b). Relational violence is often bidirectional and can quickly escalate, making it physically and emotionally damaging for both partners, though women are often more vulnerable to the consequences of physical aggression. In general, incarceration undermines the health of a relationship in many facets; those in relationships involving an incarcerated partner reported more conflict and issues when compared to those who were not dealing with the carceral system (Siennick et al., 2014). The conflict and stress stemming from a partner's incarceration often degrade relationships, as data shows higher divorce rates for those dealing with the system (Siennick et al., 2014).

There is evidence that healthy, high-quality romantic relationships are protective factors for incarcerated people. Smith et al. (2024) found that incarcerated men who were single, in neutral-quality relationships, or in poor-quality relationships reported far worse overall health and mental health than those in high-quality romantic relationships. This finding suggests there could be benefits to supporting the health of incarcerated people's romantic relationships, as folks with higher quality romantic relationships report better health than those not in high-quality relationships.

When romantic partners dealing with the carceral system find themselves in a freefall, MFTs can serve as a parachute that helps them navigate to safety. Programs that are tailored toward helping partners may be few and far between, but their impact cannot be understated. Being able to adequately support couples can reduce recidivism, reduce relational violence, improve health, decrease stress, create better parenting units to support children, and overall improve communities by fostering the love between partners rather than leaving it to corrode. A thorough search through the literature on interventions revealed just one therapy specifically targeting romantic partners, which is discussed below.

Solution-Focused Brief Couple Therapy

Solution-Focused Brief Couple Therapy (SFBCT) focuses on motivating romantic partners to solve problems through the utilization of their strengths in identifying and implementing solutions (Jalali et al., 2018). To accomplish this, therapists direct clients in identifying strengths and ways of being that have helped them meet their goals in the past so they can apply those same abilities to meet their current goals. Over the course of roughly six sessions a few goals should be establishing the therapist and client relationship, goal setting, debating problems which may get in the way of said goal setting, and planning for the future. In the past, SFBCT has struggled to prove effective; however, the intervention has been refined over the years and now is effective in improving marital satisfaction between couples dealing with the carceral system. This method is best suited for couples who need immediate results and solutions in their relationship that threaten the stability or even the existence of their relationship.

SFBCT Case Example

Mikailah (32F) and Alyssa (41F) are a couple with two young children, York (6M) and Brooklyn (8F). The stability of all of their lives is now compromised as Alyssa has been arrested for drug possession for the third time. Their family relies on each and every paycheck to survive and now Alyssa, who was the primary source of income in her family, is unable to supply financial support for her household. Mikailah now struggles to pay living expenses, so she began working a second job. Between working, domestic tasks, and caring for their kids, Mikailah has little time to visit or call Alyssa. Tension, resentment, blame, and inability to connect cause their relationship to quickly deteriorate. When Alyssa is able to reach Mikailah, Alyssa requests money for calls and items. Mikailah refuses because she is financially struggling and would prefer to direct the money toward their children. Arguments about money have dominated their conversations, and they rarely talk about intimacy, their feelings about their situation, or their plans for the future.

Considering Mikailah and Alyssa's resonation with the queer community, the supervising therapist at their facility assigned them to a student therapist who identifies as queer and non-binary. The couple's assigned therapist, Fatima, is an MFT graduate student who uses the neo-pronouns xe/xyr.

Neo-pronouns function as gender neutral alternatives to binary she/her and he/him pronouns. Fatima is interning at the prison, which is near xyr school. Fatima facilitates conversations about how recent events and their struggles at home and prison have been affecting their ability to connect with one another. Through this conversation, Fatima brings attention to what relational dynamics need improvement. Fatima challenges the couple to think about how they can prevent their struggles from continuing or reoccurring by prompting them to remember times when their communication and relationship were healthy. Fatima also asks them to describe how they coped and maintained their relationship during Alyssa's prior sentences to investigate if there were times when they were able to do so more effectively. Fatima's prompts allow the couple to reminisce on times when their approach to communication was loving and productive to highlight their ability to replicate those old approaches in their current situation. Showing them that they already have the skills to communicate effectively, highlights their resiliency and ability to adapt. Xe also encourages the couple to plan how they will prevent Alyssa from reoffending and what resources have been effective in preventing her from relapsing in the past. While Fatima cannot explicitly prevent issues, xe can provide clients with the tools to better manage any issues that arise between them in the present and future of their journey with the justice system. All of these tactics work to help Mikailah and Alyssa feel emotionally intimate and promote their ability to work as a team in coping with Alyssa's incarceration, release, and recovery.

Adults and Their Children

Approximately 648,500 incarcerated individuals, constituting half of state and federal prison populations, are parents to at least one child (Maruschak et al., 2021). Many of these parents have multiple children, leaving approximately 1.5 million children living without a parent. It is important to note that these statistics are drawn from the prison population in 2016, and the rates of incarceration grow every year. The amount of parents and children currently impacted by the federal and state prison system is likely understated in the above text.

Because children are unable to provide their incarcerated parents with a roof or a paying job post-release, they are often excluded from therapeutic interventions. There are programs that encourage parental education and visitation, such as Aid to Inmate Mothers or AIM (Denny, 2011). However, there are few programs that support parents and their children therapeutically. Nationally, there are three states with prison nurseries that offer relational therapy for the mothers and babies they house (The Rebecca Project, 2010). Overall, there are very few programs for mothers and few if any for fathers.

There are numerous negative emotions that accompany being separated from a child. The ability for incarcerated parents to support their child(ren) is source of shame, stress, loneliness, anxiety, frustration, and depression (Arditti et al., 2005; Gallegos et al., 2023; Greif, 2014; Houck & Loper, 2002; Loper et al., 2009). They worry about how impossible it is to make up for those lost childhood years and how saying congratulations in a letter or a phone call is simply not the same as being witness to someone's life and being part of their upbringing. Those first steps, recitals, games, and graduations, all spent behind bars. Having empowering and healing therapy that creates an excuse for parents and their children to come together creates opportunities for connectedness that could reduce feelings of shame and longing for incarcerated parents.

Despite the smaller role children play in reducing their parent's recidivism, the consequence of excluding them from relational therapy is that the children themselves may enter the carceral system. The emotions that accompany losing a parent are not only strong but also directly impact the development of the brain (Bowlby, 1973; Briggs-Gowan et al., 2019; Schore, 2001; Sullivan, 2012). The growing brain is extremely vulnerable to stress. Big changes such as a parent's removal from the home or being separated during infancy overwhelm children's delicate minds, inflating their sense of danger and impeding their development of healthy responses to stress. The world is so aware of the devastating effect parental separation can have on young minds that only four nations in the world forcibly separate incarcerated mothers from their newborns including the Bahamas, Liberia, Suriname, and the United States (Warner, 2015).

In the current system, children's needs are neglected, and their connection with their parents is left to deteriorate. The devastating effects of losing a parent are evident in how children of incarcerated people think and behave. If children do not receive adequate support around a parent's incarceration, they may develop attachment problems that lead to maladaptive coping strategies and disordered ways of being (Poehlmann, 2005). They are more likely to suffer mental health conditions, develop serious attachment disorders, display aggression, engage in risky sexual behaviors, engage in drug use, and fall dangerously behind their peers in educational development (Dallaire, 2007; Geller et al., 2012; Gifford et al., 2019; Haskins, 2014, 2016; Kopak & Smith-Ruiz, 2016; Margolies et al., 2006; Murray & Farrington, 2005). All of these mental and behavioral outcomes contribute to them being at higher risk of committing legal offenses that could result in them suffering the same fate as their incarcerated parents. Interventions that support Kiddos and their parents are paramount to supporting parent and child well-being and disrupting generational cycles of disadvantage by sponsoring brighter futures.

Case Example

John (28M) has been serving a 15-year sentence for armed robbery, possession, and intent to distribute. He was incarcerated five years ago. John has two children, Emma (12F) and Michael (10M). Their mom, Destiny (27F), is not present in their lives because she moved away with a different romantic partner when Emma was 3 and Micheal was 1. The kids have been living with their paternal grandparents, Sherrie and Allen, ever since John's incarceration.

Emma has been struggling with feelings of abandonment and anger, which have manifested in behavioral problems at school and withdrawal at home. She frequently claims that no one loves her and that her grandmother kidnapped her. She asks a lot of questions about her dad, who she has not had contact with since his incarceration because he lives so far away. Michael is anxious and clingy. If he is not constantly accompanied by his grandmother or sister, he has emotional outbursts and sometimes tears pictures off of walls. He texts and calls them constantly while he is at school. It is evident that both children have experienced significant emotional distress due to their father's absence. John is depressed because committed himself to raising his children by himself after Destiny left and he feels as though he has failed them. Sherrie does not help John keep in contact with Emma and Micheal. She refuses to give him their phone numbers because she believes he is verbally abusive and a bad influence.

Delanie, an MFT graduate student, is interning at a state prison by her university. She has been assigned to work with John because he requested family therapy after Sherrie called him to express concern about Emma and Micheal's behavior. Delanie's goal is to create a sense of stability and love for Emma and Micheal by reunifying and emotionally connecting them with John. Delanie's first intervention, prior to everyone seeing each other, is to facilitate an initial contact between John and his kids through an exchange of letters, where they can express their feelings without the awkwardness of handing the letter to someone who may feel like a stranger. Delanie discusses with Sherrie that she will help John write his letter with healthy expressions of his feelings, and suggests that Sherrie read the letters before giving them to the kids. Delanie works with John to alter his communication methods from contempt and aggression to vulnerability and kindness. She encourages the family to continue sending letters at least once a week, emphasizing that the letters are a physical reminder for the kids that their father is in their lives and loves them.

Because the prison is far away from their home, Delanie organizes biweekly virtual video calls for John, Emma, and Micheal. As a trauma-informed therapist, Delanie knows talk therapy is not the best approach to use with kiddos. Instead she facilitates activities where the family can express themselves through play such as role-playing exercises and art therapy. As their sessions progress and the family knows each other more, Delanie guides exercises that build love between John, Emma, and Micheal such as having each person share their favorite memory of each other, or going back and forth and describing things they love about each other. Though such activities may seem simple, they are informed by trauma and play therapy principles. These activities can be transformative in the reunification process, helping Emma and Micheal feel more heard, understood, loved, and connected with their father.

Lessons and Ideas for the Future

Thinkers from multiple disciplines: psychology, psychiatry, sociology, counseling, and criminology have offered their thoughts and ideas about what is best for incarcerated people and their families regarding relational therapeutic interventions. The following is a list of suggestions for future MFT interventions informed by moral and empirical arguments voiced throughout the existing literature.

Integrating Approaches

Historically, modern approaches to therapy have been problem-focused and directive, where therapists assume authority over a family system, identify what should change, and make suggestions about how such changes should occur. These approaches do not necessarily value the opinions or perspectives of the clients during treatment planning. Such approaches replicate the justice system by perpetuating the use of control to pathologize people and target their symptoms rather than addressing the causes of symptoms such as oppression, alienation, marginalization, and abuse. Such approaches are effective in quickly altering family dynamics and structures but do not address more deep rooted issues.

Alternatively, postmodern approaches are highly collaborative, client-specific approaches designed with intersectionality and sociocultural attunement in mind. Postmodern approaches encapsulate a recent societal paradigm shift. Rather than blaming peoples' problems on internal pathology and focusing on the problems themselves, postmodern clinicians recontextualize problems as symptoms of external dysfunction and highlight internal strengths that can be utilized to overcome issues. By externalizing problems and emphasizing the good in people, postmodern approaches center wellness and empowerment. The collaborative element of postmodern approaches is also empowering as it allows imprisoned people, arguably some of the most powerless people in the world, to have control over their treatment. Additionally, the flexibility and personalization inherent in these approaches recognize the diverse experiences and perspectives of incarcerated individuals and their families. Through collaborative and individualized treatment planning, clients' voices are heard, believed, and attuned to by their therapists. Such an experience lies in stark contrast to the structure and nature of prisons where individual power and control are stripped entirely.

Both modern and postmodern approaches can be beneficial for working with the incarcerated population as one provides structure and guidance while the other provides a space to process emotion and challenge oppression, all of which are crucial for this population, especially prior to reentry. Though the concept of amalgamating treatment models is not new, there are few guidelines on how to do so in an informed and effective manner. The Tadros theory of change is an example of how theories can be combined in a logical manner (Tadros, 2019). The theory integrates the empowering attitudes of narrative therapy, the future-focused goal orientation of solution-focused therapy, the framework of multicultural cultural therapy, and the positivity of strengths-based approaches into the foundation of SFT to create a cohesive approach that balances strictness with acceptance. Moving forward, it may benefit incarcerated people and their families to infuse strength and empowerment-based models into the modern approaches that are already being used. Such a shift in treatment approaches could possibly enhance the effectiveness of interventions and perhaps make therapy more enjoyable for clients. There are strong moral arguments supporting the implementation of two theories in particular: multicultural and trauma-informed family therapy.

Multicultural

Integration of a multicultural framework characterized by sociocultural attunement, respect for cultural differences, and the ability to discuss cultural differences in a therapeutic setting may be one of the most imperative changes needed in the field, as most of the people in prison are people of color with racially and culturally diverse systems. Those involved with the carceral system report enduring perpetual interpersonal, institutional, and societal disrespect, humiliation, and rejection (Arditti & Few, 2006, Kupers, 2005, Porgrebin et al., 2015). Using multicultural frameworks allows clinicians to hold themselves to a higher standard of attunement and be understanding of the impacts of social location and relational intersectionality on clients' lived experiences (Tadros et al., 2019; Tadros & Owens, 2021). This awareness allows clinicians to create a space where incarcerated people can experience respect, appreciation, and grace.

Trauma-Informed

Incarceration can manifest trauma through many avenues and a significant amount of incarcerated individuals have endured development and complex trauma histories prior to their incarceration. For instance, many women enter the carceral system pregnant with their abuser's or rapist's child. Regardless of individual trauma experiences, there is a universal trauma endured by everyone impacted by incarceration: grief. Incarceration can create grief for parents and grandparents of incarcerated children, children of incarcerated parents, siblings of incarcerated people, and for the incarcerated person themselves, leading to further trauma for everyone involved (Arditti, 2012; Arditti et al., 2005; Lantigua-Williams, 2016; Tadros et al., 2020). By integrating trauma-informed care into family interventions, therapists can mitigate the impact of incarceration-related and unrelated trauma on incarcerated people and their families.

Length and Context of Treatment

One of the most critical factors in the success of therapeutic interventions is the therapist-client alliance. Research consistently shows that the quality of this relationship is the greatest predictor of positive change and client satisfaction with treatment (Norcross & Lambert, 2011, 2018). Building a strong therapist-client alliance can be particularly challenging in the prison setting, where trust and attachment issues are prevalent among incarcerated individuals. Many incarcerated individuals have experienced significant trauma, leading to heightened mistrust and difficulties in forming new relationships. Developing a strong therapeutic alliance in this context could require a considerable amount of time, perhaps years, to overcome these barriers and establish a meaningful connection. Unfortunately, interventions for this population are usually brief, typically lasting no more than eight months regardless of the length of sentences.

In addition to the overall length of treatment, the context in which treatment takes place is also an area for improvement. There is a need for continuous therapeutic support that extends beyond the period of incarceration. Post-release family therapy has been effective in decreasing family contention, improving adverse mental health symptoms, increasing familial connectedness, and improving family functioning (Datchi & Sexton, 2013).

One of the most difficult ideas to implement is keeping therapists consistent. Existing programs, particularly those for juveniles, have one clinician continue treatment from a client's incarceration to the months following release. Maintaining the same therapist throughout the treatment process could aid in building strong therapist-client alliances that foster trust and rapport. A stable therapeutic relationship helps clients feel secure and supported, enhancing the overall effectiveness of the intervention.

The literature recommends that recently released parents and their children undergo reunification therapy to help them reconnect following long periods of separation (Faust, 2018; Negash et al., 2022b). For the larger family, emotion-focused family therapy and contextual family therapy may be helpful for healing familial bonds where there has been significant betrayal, trauma, and injustice (Garofalo, 2020; Landers et al., 2020). Landers et al. (2020) also recommend structural, narrative, and strategic family therapies during reentry. Overall, regardless of theory, post-release therapies help to ensure that the positive changes achieved during incarceration are sustained and that families can navigate the challenges of reintegration with ongoing professional support.

Barriers and How to Break Them

Despite evidence showing the benefits of relational therapy for individuals impacted by the carceral system, there are many barriers preventing the implementation of relational therapy. The most prevalent of them are outlined below with suggestions on how to confront them from the literature. See the subsections below.

Funding

Perhaps the largest barrier in providing care is funding. Many prisons either lack state funding or are privatized and as a result have less money to invest into the mental health care of incarcerated persons. Government funding is also an unreliable source, as the allocated funds can be revoked and redirected if new politicians are elected who have values elsewhere. Family therapy is inherently not a service that can be implemented with little to no effort and usually requires long-time investments in order to be effective.

Many institutions continue to not include MFTs among their staff, which has resulted in insufficient care for incarcerated populations and has perpetuated the ongoing lack of coverage this topic receives (Tadros et al., 2022). A lack of coverage works to reinforce barriers between clients and care as a lack of discussion means less opportunity for funding and the strengthening of stigmas. This issue is not without potential solutions though, as there are largely underutilized options which could shatter barriers stopping incarcerated individuals and their loved ones from receiving support and care. Prisons could recruit masters and PhD student interns who are working to reach thresholds of hours spent with clients in order to graduate and apply for licensure. This would be a three-way mutually beneficial arrangement, with unlicensed interns accumulating hours and experience needed for licensure, prisons acquiring free labor, and incarcerated people and their families being connected to treatment they otherwise would not have access to Barretti & Beitin (2010). Information on training and informing student interns to operate and navigate environments with incarcerated persons is thoroughly outlined in *The Experiences of Marriage and Family Therapists Working in Incarcerated Settings* (Tadros et al., 2021).

Family Involvement

Therapy as a concept is stigmatized in many cultures, leading communities to believe those who need it are weak. Such stigma can discourage people from seeking help after release, hence why exposing them to mental health care during their sentence is critical (Negash et al., 2022b). Families may teach their children that therapy is for those who suffer from mental illnesses or for those who are not strong enough to face their problems, which could lead to hesitation from certain members to participate. In order to combat stigmas, therapists can connect with pillars of support the family may already have such as school systems and religious organizations who can adequately and respectfully educate members of the community on the importance of mental health (Negash et al., 2022b).

Additionally, family members may have strong negative sentiments toward the incarcerated person that make them unwilling to reconnect with the incarcerated person or participate in family therapy. This is especially true in the case of guardians of children, usually grandparents, extended family, foster family, and current or ex-partners (Roy & Dyson, 2005). Their negative opinions of the incarcerated person may lead them to further alienate the parent trying to reconnect. Therapists could act to create bridges built of common ground and shared goals through reaching out to family members, especially guardians of children, to explain the value of reunification in the context of that particular family.

Unlocking Empathy

The research on incarcerated people's experiences is currently gendered, heteronormative, and exclusionary to people with physical disabilities. Such exclusion limits our ability to apply the efficacy of theoretical interventions to everyone in the prison system. Interventions that are not mindful of the beauty and nuance of intersectionality are a disservice to the incarcerated population who are disproportionately struggling with complex combinations of multi-marginalized identities. Queerness, Deafness, and Religiosity are among many other facets of human identity that therapists must acknowledge, accommodate, and attune to during treatment.

Incarceration is inarguably a strenuous experience for any human being, and what individuals and their families need when dealing with the carceral system is structured and tailored support informed by their unique identities, experiences, trauma, and background. This population lives in conflict with multiple systems simultaneously. Societal, institutional, and familial systems all negatively impact them to the point of desperation, mental illness, and hopelessness that traps them at their worst state of being. The therapeutic interventions offered by MFTs are inherently systemic, making them possibly the best fit for offering care to the most oppressed group of people in America.

The interventions MFTs deliver benefit not just the client but can actually have profound effects on society as a whole due to MFTs abilities to reduce rates of recidivism and increase relationship health and satisfaction. Being able to ensure a smooth reintegration into their community by creating a strong support system. In an ideal world, ample time and resources would be invested in the staffing of MFTs and the implementation of their programs. However, economic and moral restraints limit the ability for government facilities to invest in the well-being of the humans they house. There are multiple options for increasing the presence of MFTs and MFT interventions in carceral settings without overreliance on government funding and investments. Facilities could recruit interns from masters programs or host multi-family group therapies with the employment of just a few extra staff. With the cost of crime, such an investment into decreasing recidivism, supporting improved well-being, and disrupting generational cycles would surely be worth the extra salaries.

Netflix's recent documentary, *Unlocked: A Jail Experiment*, became one of the platform's most-watched shows in 2024, conveying that the need for prison reform is entering the mainstream consciousness (Higgins, 2024). It was obvious the cast were suffering from their social isolation and forced alienation on part of the Pulaski County Regional Detention Facility and how something as simple as allowing them to call their families transformed their well-being. As society begins to acknowledge the dichotomy of privilege and oppression, it is paramount that we unite to humanize, platform, support, and advocate for the 1 in 100 Americans behind bars and the millions of people who miss them. It would be a disservice to humanity if the recent mental health movement that sparked the trend of prioritizing mental prosperity and de-stigmatizing psychological impairments did not extend to the most stressed, traumatized, and isolated populations among us. Relational therapy could help them connect with home when they need it most so that one day they can return to their place of residence and stay there.

References

Andrews, D. A., & Bonta, J. (2010). The empirical base of PCC and the RNR model of assessment and crime prevention through human service. In E. S. Boyne (Ed.), *The psychology of criminal conduct* (5th ed., pp. 45–78). LexisNexis.

Aos, S. (2004). *Washington State's family integrated transitions program for juvenile offenders: Outcome evaluation and benefit-cost analysis.* Olympia: Washington State Institute for Public Policy.

Arditti, J. A. (2012). Child trauma within the context of parental incarceration: A family process perspective. *Journal of Family Theory & Review*, *4*(3), 181–219. https://doi.org/10.1111/j.1756-2589.2012.00128.x

Arditti, J. A., & Few, A. L. (2006). Mothers' reentry into family life following incarceration. *Criminal Justice Policy Review, 17*(1), 103–123. https://doi.org/10.1177/0887403405282450

Arditti, J., Jordan S. S., & Parkman, T. (2005). "It's been hard to be a father": A qualitative exploration of incarcerated fatherhood. *Fathering, 3*(3), 267–288. https://doi.org/10.3149/fth.0303.267.

Bales, W., & Mears, D. (2008). Inmate social ties and the transition to society: Does visitation reduce recidivism? *Journal of Research in Crime and Delinquency, 45*(3), 287–321. https://doi.org/10.1177/0022427808317574.

Barretti, L. M., & Beitin, B. K. (2010). Creating internships in marriage and family therapy: A collaboration between a training program and an offender reentry facility. *Contemporary Family Therapy: An International Journal, 32*(1), 39–51. https://doi.org/10.1007/s10591-009-9109-3

Basto-Pereira, M., Gouveia-Pereira, M., Pereira, C. R., Barrett, E. L., Lawler S., Newton, N., Stapinski, L., Prior, K., Costa, M. S. A., Ximenes, J. M., Rocha, A. S., Michel, G., Garcia, M., Rouchy, E., Al Shawi, A., Sarhan, Y., Fulano, C., Magaiam, A. J., El-Astal, S., & Sakulku, J. (2022). The global impact of adverse childhood experiences on criminal behavior: A cross-continental study. *Child Abuse & Neglect*. Advance online publication. 124, 105459. https://doi.org/10.1016/j.chiabu.2021.105459

Bowlby, J. (1973). *Attachment and loss: Separation: Anxiety and anger. (Vol. 2)*. New York: Basic Books.

Briggs-Gowan, M. J., Greene, C., Ford, J., Clark, R., McCarthy, K. J., & Carter, A. S. (2019). Adverse impact of multiple separations or loss of primary caregivers on young children. *European Journal of Psychotraumatology, 10*(1), 1646965. https://doi.org/10.1080/20008198.2019.1646965

Butler, L., & Taylor, E. (2022). A second chance: The impact of unsuccessful reentry and the need for reintegration resources in communities. *Community Policing Dispatch, 15*(4). https://cops.usdoj.gov/html/dispatch/04-2022/reintegration_resources.html

Celinska, K., College, J., York, N., Furrer, S., & Cheng, C. (2013). An outcome-based evaluation of functional family therapy for youth with behavioral problems. *Journal of Juvenile Justice, 2*(2), 23–36.

Clark, V. A., & Duwe, G. (2017). Distance matters: Examining the factors that impact prisoner visitation in Minnesota. *Criminal Justice and Behavior, 44*(2), 184–204. https://doi.org/10.1177/0093854816667416

Cochran, J. C., Mears, D. P., Bales, W. D., & Stewart, E. A. (2016). Spatial distance, community disadvantage, and racial and ethnic variation in prison inmate access to social ties. *Journal of Research in Crime and Delinquency, 53*(2), 220–254. https://doi.org/10.1177/0022427815592675

Comfort, M., McKay, T., Landwehr, J., Kennedy, E., Lindquist, C., & Bir, A. (2016). The costs of incarceration for families of prisoners. *International Review of the Red Cross, 98*(3), 783–798. https://doi.org/2443/10.1017/S1816383117000704

Dallaire, D. H. (2007). Children with incarcerated mothers: Developmental outcomes, special challenges and recommendations. *Journal of Applied Developmental Psychology, 28*(1), 15–24. https://doi.org/10.1016/j.appdev.2006.10.003

Daniel, A. E. (2007). Care of the mentally ill in prisons: Challenges and solutions. *Journal of the American Academy of Psychiatry and the Law Online*, *35*(4), 406–410. PMID: 18086729

Datchi, C. C., Barretti, L. M., & Thompson, C. M. (2016). Family services in adult detention centers: Systemic principles for prisoner reentry. *Couple and Family Psychology: Research and Practice*, *5*(2), 89–104. https://doi.org/10.1037/cfp0000057

Datchi, C. C., & Sexton, T. L. (2013). Can family therapy have an effect on adult criminal conduct? Initial evaluation of functional family therapy. *Couple and Family Psychology: Research and Practice*, *2*(4), 278–293. https://doi.org/10.1037/a0034166

Denney, A. S., Tewksbury, R., & Jones, R. S. (2014). Beyond basic needs: Social support and structure for successful offender reentry. *Journal of Qualitative Criminal Justice & Criminology*. *2*(1), 39–67. https://doi.org/10.21428/88de04a1.d95029f6

Denny, J. (2011). Spotlight on: aid to inmate mothers. *Children's Legal Rights Journal*, *31*(1), 56–93.

Durante, K. A., Phillips Meertins, J. R., & Tadros, E. (2024). Institutional relational maintenance barriers and perceptions of relationship quality among women with incarcerated partners. *Crime & Delinquency*, *70*(3), 788–811. Advance online publication. https://doi-org/10.1177/0011128722

Dutcher, T., & Barnes-Ceeney, K. (2021). Facing the ties that bind: Understanding experiences of men with an incarcerated romantic partner. *International Journal of Offender Therapy and Comparative Criminology*, *67*(10–11), 999–1016. https://doi.org/10.1177/0306624X211059319

Elderbroom, B., Bennett, L., Gong, S., Rose, F., & Towns, Z. (2018). Every second: The impact of the incarceration crisis on America's families. FWD.us. https://everysecond.fwd.us/downloads/everysecond.fwd.us.pdf

Faust, J. (2018). *Reunification family therapy: A treatment manual*. Hogrefe Publishing.

First Step Alliance. (2022). Rehabilitation lessons from Norway's prison system. *First Step Alliance*. https://www.firststepalliance.org/post/norway-prison-system-lessons

Folk, J. B., Stuewig, J., Mashek, D., Tangney, J. P., & Grossmann, J. (2019). Behind bars but connected to family: Evidence for the benefits of family contact during incarceration. *Journal of Family Psychology*, *33*(4), 453–464. https://doi.org/10.1037/fam0000520

Fulcher, P. A. (2013). The double-edged sword of prison video visitation: Claiming to keep families together while furthering the aims of the prison industrial complex. *Florida A&M University Law Review*, *9*(1), 83–112. ISSN: 1935–5173 https://commons.law.famu.edu/famulawreview/vol9/iss1/5

Gallegos, M. L., Segrin, C., & Thompson, A. (2023). Parent-child relationships and the health of incarcerated mothers: Exploring the mediating role of loneliness. *Health Communication*, *38*(7), 1442–1453. https://doi.org/10.1080/10410236.2021.2012014

Garofalo, M. (2020). Family therapy in corrections: Implications for reentry into the community. *Journal of Correctional Health Care*, *26*(3), 240–248. https://doi.org/10.1177/1078345820938350

Geller, A., Cooper, C. E., Garfinkel, I., Schwartz-Soicher, O., & Mincy, R. B. (2012). Beyond absenteeism: Father incarceration and child development. *Demography*, *49*(1), 49–76. https://doi.org/10.1007/s13524-011-0081-9

Geller, A., Garfinkel, I., Cooper, C. E., & Mincy, R. B. (2009). Parental incarceration and child well-being: Implications for urban families. *Social Science Quarterly*, *90*(5), 1186–1202. https://www.jstor.org/stable/42940627

Gifford, E. J., Eldred Kozecke, L., Golonka, M., Hill, S. N., Costello, E. J., Shanahan, L., & Copeland, W. E. (2019). Association of parental incarceration with psychiatric and functional outcomes of young adults. *JAMA Network Open*, *2*(8), e1910005–e1910005. https://doi.org/10.1001/jamanetworkopen.2019.10005

Goodey, S., Spuhler, B., & Bradford, K. (2019). Relationship education among incarcerated populations. *Marriage & Family Review*, *55*(7), 651–666. https://doi.org/10.1080/01494929.2019.1589615

Greif, G. L. (2014). The voices of fathers in prison: Implications for family practice. *Journal of Family Social Work*, *17*(1), 68–80. https://doi.org/10.1080/10522158.2013.865284

Hartnett, D., Carr, A., Hamilton, E., & O'Reilly, G. (2017). The effectiveness of functional family therapy for adolescent behavioral and substance misuse problems: A meta-analysis. *Family Process*, *56*(3), 607–619. https://doi.org/10.1111/famp.12256

Haskins, A. R. (2014). Unintended consequences: Effects of paternal incarceration on child school readiness and later special education placement. *Sociological Science*, *1*(11), 141–158. https://doi.org/10.15195/v1.a11houck

Haskins, A. R. (2016). Beyond boys' bad behavior: Paternal incarceration and cognitive development in middle childhood. *Social Forces*, *95*(2), 861–892. https://doi.org/10.1093/sf/sow066

Henggeler, S. W., Melton, G. B., & Smith, L. A. (1992). Family preservation using multisystemic therapy: An effective alternative to incarcerating serious juvenile offenders. *Journal of Consulting and Clinical Psychology*, *60*(6), 953–961. https://doi.org/10.1037/0022-006X.60.6.953

Henggeler, S. W., & Schaeffer, C. M. (2016). Multisystemic therapy®: Clinical overview, outcomes, and implementation research. *Family Process*, *55*(3), 514–528. https://doi.org/10.1111/famp.12232

Higgins, E. (Project Director). (2024, April 10). In C. Aguilar, J. C. Begley, G. Henry, I. Holub, G. Kralovansky, M. Weber, K. Woodard (Executive Producers), *Unlocked: A jail experiment*. Lucky 8.

Houck, K. D. F., & Loper, A. B. (2002). The relationship of parenting stress to adjustment among mothers in prison. *American Journal of Orthopsychiatry*, *72*(4), 548–558. https://doi.org/10.1037//0002-9432.72.4.548

Jalali, F., Hashemi, S., Kimiaei, S., Hasani, A., & Jalali, M. (2018). The effectiveness of solution-focused brief couple therapy on marital satisfaction among married prisoners and their wives. *International Journal of Offender Therapy and Comparative Criminology*, *62*(10), 3023–3037. https://doi.org/10.1177/0306624X17733662

Keiley, M. K. (2007). Multiple-family group intervention for incarcerated adolescents and their families: A pilot project. *Journal of Marital and Family Therapy*, *33*(1), 106–124. https://doi-org/10.1111/j.1752-0606.2007.00009.x

Kopak, A. M., & Smith-Ruiz, D. (2016). Criminal justice involvement, drug use, and depression among African American children of incarcerated parents. *Race and Justice*, *6*(2), 89–116. https://doi-org/10.1177/2153368715586633

Kupers, T. A. (2005). Toxic masculinity as a barrier to mental health treatment in prison. *Journal of Clinical Psychology*, *61*(6), 713–724. https://doi.org/10.1002/jclp.20105

Landers, A., Simpson, J., Gagner, N., & Robinson, B. (2020, November 12). *Beyond borders: Reunifying families in family therapy* [Conference presentation]. AAMFT 2020 Annual Conference.

Lantigua-Williams, J. (2016, November, 18). Losing your brothers to prison. *The Atlantic*. https://www.theatlantic.com/national/archive/2016/11/the-brothers-i-once-knew-have-died/622726/

Liddle, H. A. (2014). Adapting and implementing an evidence-based treatment with justice-involved adolescents: The example of multidimensional family therapy. *Family Process*, *53*(3), 516–528. https://doi.org/10.1111/famp.12094

Liddle, H. A., Dakof, G., Rowe, C., Mohamed, A. B., Henderson, C., Foulkrod, T., Lucas, M., & DiFrancesco, M. (2024). Multidimensional family therapy for justice-involved young adults with substance use disorders. *The Journal of Behavioral Health Services & Research*, *51*(2), 250–263. https://doi.org/10.1007/s11414-023-09852-5

Lindforss, L., & Magnusson, D. (1997). Solution-focused therapy in prison. *Contemporary Family Therapy*, *19*(1), 89–103. https://doi.org/10.1023/A:1026114501186

Liu, L., & Visher, C. A. (2021). Decomposition of the role of family in reentry: Family support, tension, gender, and reentry outcomes. *Crime & Delinquency*, *67*(6–7), 970–996. https://doi.org/10.1177/0011128720987195

Loeber, R., Farrington, D. P., & Petechuk, D. (2013). *Bulletin 1: From juvenile delinquency to young adult offending (Study group on the transitions between juvenile delinquency and adult crime)* (NCJ No. 242931). U.S. Department of Justice. National Criminal Justice Reference Service. https://www.ncjrs.gov/pdffiles1/nij/grants/242931.pdf

Loper, A. B., Carlson, L. W., Levitt, L., & Scheffel, K. (2009). Parenting stress, alliance, child contact, and adjustment of imprisoned mothers and fathers. *Journal of Offender Rehabilitation*, *48*(6), 483–503. https://doi.org/10.1080/10509670903081300

Margolies, J. K., & Kraft-Stolar, T. (2006). *When "free" means losing your mother: The collision of child welfare and the incarceration of women in New York State*. Correctional Association of New York. https://repositories.lib.utexas.edu/bitstream/handle/2152/15159/When_Free_Rpt_Feb_2006.pdf?sequence=2&isAllowed=y

Martha Wright-Reed Just and Reasonable Communications Act of 2022, Pub. L. No. 117–338 (2022). U.S. Government Publishing Office. https://www.congress.gov/bill/117th-congress/senate-bill/1541/text

Maruschak, L. M., Bronson, J., & Alper, M. (2021). *Parents in prison and their minor children: Survey of prison inmates, 2016*. Bureau of Justice Statistics, Office of Justice Programs. U.S. Department of Justice. https://bjs.ojp.gov/content/pub/pdf/pptmcspi16st.pdf.

McKay, T., Comfort, M., Grove, L., Bir, A., & Lindquist, C. (2018a). Whose punishment, whose crime? Understanding parenting and partnership in a time of mass incarceration. *Journal of Offender Rehabilitation*, *57*(2), 69–82. https://doi.org/10.1080/10509674.2017.1294640

McKay, T., Comfort, M., Lindquist, C., & Bir, A. (2016). If family matters: Supporting family relationships during incarceration and reentry. *Criminology & Public Policy*, *15*(2), 529–542. https://doi.org/10.1111/1745-9133.12209

McKay, T., Landwehr, J. G., Lindquist, C., Feinberg, R. K., Comfort, M., Cohen, J., & Bir, A. (2018b). Intimate partner violence in couples navigating incarceration and reentry. *Journal of Offender Rehabilitation*, *57*(5), 273–293. https://doi.org/10.1080/10509674.2018.1487897

Murray, J., & Farrington, D. P. (2005). Parental imprisonment: Effects on boys' antisocial behavior and delinquency through the life-course. *Journal of Child Psychology and Psychiatry*, *46*(12), 1269–1278. https://doi.org/10.1111/j.1469–7610.2005.01433.x

Naser, R. L., & Visher, C. A. (2006). Family members' experiences with incarceration and reentry. *Western Criminology Review*, *7*(2), 20–31.

Negash, S., Roberson, P. N. E., Tadros, E., & DeJesus, S. Y. (2022a). A brief relationship education pilot intervention for men post release. *The Prison Journal*, *102*(3), 347–366. https://doi.org/10.1177/00328855221095560

Negash, S., Chung, K., & Oh, S. (2022b). Families post-release: Barriers and pathways to family therapy. *Family Process*, *61*(2), 609–624. https://doi.org/10.1111/famp.12769

Norcross, J. C., & Lambert, M. J. (2011). Psychotherapy relationships that work II. *Psychotherapy*, *48*(1), 4–8. https://doi.org/10.1037/a0022180

Norcross, J. C., & Lambert, M. J. (2018). Psychotherapy relationships that work III. *Psychotherapy*, *55*(4), 303–315. https://doi.org/10.1037/pst0000193

Poehlmann, J. (2005). Representations of attachment relationships in children of incarcerated mothers. *Child development*, *76*(3), 679–696. https://doi.org/10.1111/j.1467-8624.2005.00871.

Pogrebin, M. R., Stretesky, P. B., Walker, A., & Opsal, T. (2015). Rejection, humiliation, and parole: A study of parolees' perspectives. *Symbolic Interaction*, *38*(3), 413–430. https://doi.org/10.1002/symb.164

Roy, K. M., & Dyson, O. L. (2005). Gatekeeping in context: Babymama drama and the involvement of incarcerated fathers. *Fathering: A Journal of Theory, Research, and Practice about Men as Fathers*, *3*(3), 289–310. https://doi.org/10.3149/fth.0303.289

Rubenstein, B. Y., Toman, E. L., & Cochran, J. C. (2021). Socioeconomic barriers to child contact with incarcerated parents. *Justice Quarterly*, *38*(4), 725–751. https://doi.org/10.1080/07418825.2019.1606270

Schore, A. N. (2001). The effects of early relational trauma on right brain development, affect regulation, and infant mental health. *Infant Mental Health Journal*, *22*(1–2), 201–269. https://doi.org/10.1002/1097-0355(200101/04)22:1<201::AID-IMHJ8>3.0.CO;2–9

Sexton, T. L., & Alexander, J. F. (2000). *Functional family therapy*. US Department of Justice, Office of Justice Programs, Office of Juvenile Justice and Delinquency Prevention.

Sexton, T., & Turner, C. W. (2010). The effectiveness of functional family therapy for youth with behavioral problems in a community practice setting. *Journal of Family*

Psychology: JFP: Journal of the Division of Family Psychology of the American Psychological Association (Division 43), *24*(3), 339–348. https://doi.org/10.1037/a0019406

Sexton, T. L. (2016). Incarceration as a family affair: Thinking beyond the individual. *Couple and Family Psychology: Research and Practice*, *5*(2), 61–64. https://doi.org/10.1037/cfp0000062

Siennick, S. E., Stewart, E. A., & Staff, J. (2014). Explaining the association between incarceration and divorce. *Criminology: An Interdisciplinary Journal*, *52*(3), 371–398. https://doi.org/10.1111/1745-9125.12040

Silk, S., & Goldman, B. (2013). How not to say the wrong thing. *Los Angeles Times*. https://www.latimes.com/opinion/op-ed/la-xpm-2013-apr-07-la-oe-0407-silk-ringtheory-20130407-story.html

Simons, I., Mulder, E., Breuk, R., Mos, K., Rigter, H., van Domburgh, L., & Vermeiren, R. (2017). A program of family-centered care for adolescents in short-term stay groups of juvenile justice institutions. *Child and Adolescent Psychiatry and Mental Health*, *11*, 1–8. https://doi.org/10.1186/s13034-017-0203-2

Smith, C. D. IV, Riano, N. S., Randolph, I. S., Beardslee, J., & Cauffman, E. E. (2024). The panacea that is love: The influence of romantic relationships on justice-involved young adults' self-reported health. *Couple and Family Psychology: Research and Practice*. Advance online publication. https://doi.org/10.1037/cfp0000263

Sullivan, R. M. (2012). The neurobiology of attachment to nurturing and abusive caregivers. *The Hastings Law Journal*, *63*(6), 1553–1570. PMID: 24049190

Szapocznik, J., Schwartz, S. J., Muir, J. A., & Brown, C. H. (2012). Brief strategic family therapy: An intervention to reduce adolescent risk behavior. *Couple and Family Psychology: Research and Practice*, *1*(2), 134–145. https://doi.org/10.1037/a0029002

Szapocznik J., & Williams R. A. (2000). Brief strategic family therapy: Twenty-five years of interplay among theory, research and practice in adolescent behavior problems and drug abuse. *Clinical Child and Family Psychology Review*, *3*(2), 117–134. https://doi.org/10.1023/A:1009512719808

Tadros, E. (2019). The Tadros theory of change: An integrated structural, narrative, and solution-focused approach. *Contemporary Family Therapy*, *41*(4), 347–356. https://doi.org/10.1007/s10591-019-09502-z

Tadros, E., & Finney, N. (2018). Structural family therapy with incarcerated families: A clinical case study. *The Family Journal*, *26*(2), 253–261. https://doi.org/10.1177/1066480718777409

Tadros, E., & Finney, N. (2019). Exploring the utilization of structural and medical family therapy with an incarcerated mother living with HIV. *International Journal of Offender Therapy and Comparative Criminology*, *63*(4), 624–640. https://doi.org/10.1177/0306624X18821825

Tadros, E., Fye, J. M., McCrone, C. L., & Finney, N. (2019). Incorporating multicultural couple and family therapy into incarcerated settings. *International Journal of Offender Therapy and Comparative Criminology*, *63*(4), 641–658. https://doi.org/10.1177/0306624X18823442

Tadros, E., Fye, J., & Ray, A. (2020). The lived experience of sisters with an incarcerated brother: A phenomenological study. *International Journal of*

Offender Therapy and Comparative Criminology, 64(4), 335–354. https://doi.org/10.1177/0306624X19877598

Tadros, E., Hutcherson, R., & Aguirre, N. (2022). How is family therapy discussed in the literature on incarceration?: A systematic review. *The American Journal of Family Therapy, 51*(5), 673–691. https://doi.org/10.1080/01926187.2022.2031343

Tadros, E., Negron-Hobson, S., & Monterroso, E. (2024). Structural family therapy and culturally informed care with an incarcerated family: A clinical case study. *Applied Family Therapy Journal, 5*(5), 11–18.https://dx. doi.org/10.61838/kman.aftj.5.5.2

Tadros, E., & Owens, D. (2021). Clinical implications for culturally informed counseling with incarcerated individuals. *The American Journal of Family Therapy, 49*(4), 344–355. https://doi.org/10.1080/01926187.2020.1813659

Tadros, E., Schleidan, C., Jenkins, L., & Aguirre, N. (2021). The experiences of marriage and family therapists working in incarcerated settings. *The American Journal of Family Therapy, 49*(5), 461–479. https://doi.org/10.1080/01926187.2020.1834469

The Legal Aid Society. (2024, January 5). What you need to know about prison visitation. *The Legal Aid Society.* https://legalaidnyc.org/get-help/bail-incarceration/what-you-need-to-know-about-prison-visitation/#:~:text=People%20incarcerated%20before%20trial%20are

The Rebecca Project. (2010). Mothers behind bars: *A state-by-state report card and analysis of federal policies on conditions of confinement for pregnant and parenting women and the effect on their children.* Washington, DC: National Women's Law Center. https://nwlc.org/wp-content/uploads/2015/08/mothersbehindbars2010.pdf

Turney, K., Malae, K. R., Christensen, M. A., & Halpern-Meekin, S. (2023). "Even though we're married, I'm single": The meaning of jail incarceration in romantic relationships. *Criminology, 61*, 795–822. https://doi.org/10.1111/1745-9125.12349

U.S. Department of Justice, Federal Bureau of Prisons. (2019). *Inmate security designation and custody classification* (Change Notice OPI: CPD/CPB No. 5100.08, CN–1). https://www.bop.gov/policy/progstat/5100_008cn.pdf

United States Sentencing Commission. (2021). *Quick facts: Federal offenders in prison.* https://www.ussc.gov/research/quick-facts/individuals-federal-bureau-prisons

Vera Institute of Justice Family Justice Program. (2011). *Why ask about family? A guide for corrections.* Vera Institute of Justice. https://www.vera.org/downloads/publications/Why-ask-about-family-Final.pdf

Wagner, P., & Bertram, W. (2022, December). *State of phone justice 2022: The problem, the progress, and what's next.* Prison Policy Initiative. https://www.prisonpolicy.org/phones/state_of_phone_justice_2022.html

Warner, J. (2015). Infants in orange: An international model-based approach to prison nurseries. *Hastings Women's Law Journal, 26*(1), 65–92.

Wildeman, C., Lee, H., & Comfort, M. (2013). A new vulnerable population? The health of female partners of men recently released from prison. *Women's Health Issues, 23*(6), e335–e340. https://doi.org/10.1016/j.whi.2013.07.006

Chapter 6

Working with LGBTQ+ Incarcerated Individuals and Their Families

Shannon Pedersen and Jixuan Zhao

Introduction

This chapter will review literature and research on key issues, clinical needs, treatment, and systemic policies related to LGBTQ+ adults who are incarcerated, along with the impact on their relationships with partners and families. As of 2022, there are an estimated 130,000 self-identifying lesbian, gay, bisexual, and transgender adults in U.S. prisons and jails (Ghandnoosh & Stammen, 2022). First, we will discuss key issues that are situational or circumstantial to being LGBT and incarcerated, such as sexual assault rates, hormone replacement therapy (HRT), and living assignments. Then, we will review the clinical needs of this population, focused on trauma, anxiety, depression, gender dysphoria, and family and couple relationships. Last but certainly not least, we will review mental health treatment and prison policy recommendations, including limitations, to address the key issues and clinical needs. Throughout the chapter, we have included a fictional case study example to prompt questions related to these challenges and treatment recommendations.

Key Issues

Situational and Circumstantial

Within a prison or jail, there are situations and circumstances that any incarcerated individual encounters ranging from a small nuisance to life-threatening. For LGBT individuals, three primary concerns span the literature: sexual harassment and assault, access to Hormone Replacement Therapy (HRT), and living assignments. These concerns are situational and circumstantial, because even if there are policies on such matters, there are few resources and little oversight for proper implementation.

DOI: 10.4324/9781003542940-6

Federal Prison Rape Elimination Act

In September 2003, the Federal Prison Rape Elimination Act (PREA) was signed into law with the goal to eliminate sexual abuse in all types of correctional facilities (National PREA Resource Center, n.d.). While PREA does offer protections for vulnerable people and financial penalties for noncompliance, it is not enforceable with a lawsuit in court. However, one can file a lawsuit based on the 8th amendment with a precedent in Farmer v. Brennan (Lambda Legal, n.d.), particularly for issues of placement (see more below). PREA is a great example of good intent, but with a lack of resources, there are poor opportunities for meaningful follow-through.

Sexual Harassment and Assault

There are multiple reports on the issue of sexual harassment and assault in prisons and jails across the U.S., and only a select few that highlight greater concerns for LGBTQ+ incarcerated individuals. In one California prison, approximately two-thirds LGBTQ+ incarcerated individuals reported sexual assault while incarcerated (Dolovich, 2011). Issues of harassment and assault occur in two primary contexts—between those who are incarcerated and those from staff. In both cases, there are widespread issues of physical and sexual abuse and humiliation, with transgender women and lesbians facing the greatest risks. It is important to note a common narrative that lesbian women are sexual predators in prison, but research shows they are at a higher risk of harassment and sexual abuse by peers, and even more so by male staff and correctional officers who seek to "change her mind" (Cammett, 2009).

In peer contexts, there is a wide range of accounts of abuse by fellow incarcerated individuals. Often, harassment and assault are evident through inappropriate remarks and verbal harassment. However, there are also exceptional issues of physical sexual assault and rape. One example includes forced prostitution by a correctional officer (CO) to other incarcerated individuals (Bassichis, 2007). In instances of rape, staff often fail to follow through with consequences for the perpetrator or simply state that claims cannot be corroborated, and rape kits are not provided.

When considering interactions between those who are incarcerated and staff, there are additional issues with searches that are often unnecessary, frisky, and abusive (Bassichis, 2007). When incarcerated individuals attempt to report their experiences, they typically encounter a lack of accountability for correctional officers and might also experience retaliation from COs, other staff, or their peers. While all of the above issues are present outside of a prison or jail, it is critical to note the exceptionally higher rates for those who are at the intersection of being incarcerated and LGBT.

Hormone Replacement Therapy (HRT)

In addition to general mistreatment and abuse, there is rampant denial of medical and mental health care, particularly for transgender and nonbinary individuals accessing hormones for hormone replacement therapy (HRT) and other transition-related treatments. In the 2022 U.S. Transgender Survey, 98% of respondents (over 82,000 transgender adults) on HRT reported that receiving hormones for their gender identity or transition made them more satisfied with their life (James et al., 2024). This statistic is critically tied to gender dysphoria and other mental health diagnoses, such as depression. The lack of HRT-related care while incarcerated is often due to certain facilities requiring a diagnosis and documentation of hormones and treatment *prior to* being incarcerated to receive care in the prison (Bassichis, 2007).

Outside of incarceration, the 2015 U.S. Transgender Survey reported 78% of respondents wanted to receive HRT, but only 49% of respondents had ever received it (James et al., 2016). This discrepancy can be related to financial restraints, a lack of health insurance, and inadequate access to affirmative medical professionals. For transgender or nonbinary individuals who are already on HRT prior to incarceration and are forced to discontinue use, the changes can reverse as well as negatively impact mental health. Depending on which hormones and how rapidly they are discontinued, it can also cause a form of withdrawal, which mimics menopause (Hodshire, 2023). The ramifications of discontinuing HRT for any duration while incarcerated are incredibly concerning for both mental and physical well-being purposes.

Living Assignments

Incarcerated populations are typically segregated by gender upon entering the system. Generally speaking, there are two branches of options for living assignments—being assigned by one's gender at birth versus present-day gender identity and general population versus protective custody. Both choices bring their own nuances, which often need to be considered closely in specific contexts.

Gender Assignment For those who are assigned by their sex at birth, the biggest concerns besides the aforementioned assault and harassment include issues with showers, a lack of privacy, and conflicts with appearance regulations (Bassichis, 2007). Transgender women are typically placed in men's facilities, where they are targeted by peers and correctional officers who refuse to recognize their gender identity (White Hughto et al., 2018). Transgender men do not face as much similar physical violence as transgender women, but rather more psychological oppression from the guards in the form of strip-searches and withholding hormones.

In American society, gender is inherently expressed through appearances. Unfortunately, incarcerated transgender individuals encounter disproportionate and unnecessary punishments for things such as a transgender woman being in possession of a bra because she was living in a men's prison (Bassichis, 2007). A denial of gender expression through things such as wearing bras and/or certain types of underwear, growing hair longer, and painted or longer nails for transgender women in men's prisons can perpetuate issues of gender identity and gender dysphoria, further negatively impacting other mental health diagnoses.

Protective Custody Oftentimes, solitary confinement or segregation is utilized to "contain" transgender individuals, as they don't neatly fit into one assignment and set of gendered policies. General population versus protective custody for transgender individuals is a contentious issue (Cammett, 2009). In reality, someone can be placed in protective custody for a variety of reasons. Most relevant for those who are LGBTQ+ is utilizing protective custody for those who are at a higher risk of violence or harassment by other incarcerated individuals. While the intent of this may sound beneficial on paper, the implementation and impact vary. For example, the level of safety and degree of separateness vary across facilities. This means that at one facility, protective custody could provide genuine, desired protection from other incarcerated individuals. However, it can also isolate them to an unhelpful degree, such as with solitary confinement, or put them at higher risk of harassment and abuse by correctional officers at a different facility.

Case Study

Azul is a 28-year-old Hispanic, nonbinary (assigned female at birth), queer individual who is incarcerated for theft. The theft was classified as petty theft related to survival needs, motivated by houselessness. Azul's family members include her mother, Maria (45), who was a teen mom and is a single parent, as her father died from complications of untreated diabetes. Azul has two younger siblings (15 and 20 years old) living with extended family due to housing instability. They do not currently have a significant other but are close with their family members.

As someone who is nonbinary, Azul does not neatly fit into the binary gendered incarceration system. They live in Texas, which does not allow those who are incarcerated to choose their housing assignments. Therefore, they were assigned to be with women, per their assigned sex at birth. Azul declined protective custody, as they knew the risk of solitary confinement could be more damaging than whatever harassment they might face.

Azul is also at an increased risk of sexual harassment and assault with both peers and staff while incarcerated. As someone who is nonbinary and presents more androgynous, they are harassed for being neither feminine nor masculine enough to be sexually appealing. However, this does not stop sexual assault from a Correctional Officer. Due to lack of resources, there is no recourse for the CO.

Furthermore, Azul does not have access to hormone replacement therapy, as they did not have resources to see a doctor or get a prescription prior to being incarcerated. This perpetuates gender dysphoria and the narrative that Azul is not "passing" enough as nonbinary, further complicating other mental health diagnoses.

LGBTQ+ Incarceration and the Law

While the above issues are specific to being incarcerated, there are also broader issues with LGBTQ+ encounters with the justice system that play into these concerns. The Williams Institute, a think tank at UCLA Law specializing in Sexual Orientation and Gender Identity Law and Public Policy, analyzed data from the National Inmate Survey (2012) and found that LGBTQ+ youth and adults are significantly overrepresented in the U.S. criminal justice system. Data from 2011 to 2012 revealed that individuals identifying as LGBTQ+ were incarcerated at a rate of 1,882 per 100,000 people—more than three times the national average (Srivastava et al., 2023). This disparity was largely driven by the disproportionately high incarceration rates among gay and bisexual women, whose rates were 8 to 10 times higher than the national baseline, comprising 33% of the prison population and 26.4% of those in jails (Meyer et al., 2017). In contrast, the incarceration rate for gay or bisexual men in prisons and jails was 5.5% and 3.3%, respectively, which is closer to the national average of 3.6% (Meyer et al., 2017).

Additionally, data on the transgender population reveals that nearly 17% of transgender individuals in the U.S. have been incarcerated at some point in their lives, with about 1 in 20 currently or formerly incarcerated, according to the Bureau of Justice Statistics (McCauley & Brinkley-Rubinstein, 2017). Research also indicates that LGBTQ+ youth face significantly higher rates of incarceration compared to their representation in the general population. Despite accounting for only 5–8% of the overall U.S. youth population, approximately 12–20% of those in juvenile detention facilities identify as LGBTQ+ (McCauley & Brinkley-Rubinstein, 2017). This data show that similar to other marginalized communities, LGBTQ+ individuals face an elevated risk of incarceration, often due to systemic inequalities and discrimination.

Clinical Needs

Furthermore, there are numerous clinical needs for LGBTQ+ incarcerated individuals that must be recognized and addressed. These needs encompass mental health diagnoses, trauma histories, and the complex intersection of these concerns. One critical factor is understanding the profound impact of being a minority. According to the Minority Stress Model, individuals who identify as minorities and experience discrimination or pathologization often internalize negative societal views. For this population, internalization can lead to suffering from homophobia and/or transphobia and exacerbate various mental health challenges (Frost & Meyer, 2009). As a result, these individuals may encounter traumatic or victimizing events that reinforce their fears and foster a deep mistrust of others and society (Meyer et al., 2021). The cyclical nature of victimization and trauma can directly and indirectly contribute to institutionalization and incarceration (McCauley & Brinkley-Rubinstein, 2017). Additionally, intersectional identities such as being a racial minority and queer often have a negative multiplication effect on mental health symptoms (Khan et al., 2017). Addressing these clinical needs is essential to breaking this cycle and improving mental health outcomes for LGBTQ+ individuals within the criminal justice system.

Mental Health

In the general population, LGBTQ+ people have higher rates of mental health diagnoses, particularly for mood, anxiety, and substance use disorders (Gmelin et al., 2022). Research found that incarcerated individuals who identify as lesbian and gay have a 27%-59% higher prevalence of mental health issues than heterosexual adults (Srivastava et al., 2023). Additionally, incarcerated individuals who identify as lesbian, gay and bisexual reported higher prevalence of anxiety (42%), Post-Traumatic Stress Disorder (PTSD) (71%), and manic disorder (57%) than heterosexual adults (Srivastava et al., 2023). While there are a variety of reasons for this elevated prevalence that can be attributed to factors prior to and during incarceration, it is important to note that PTSD can be exacerbated by other mental health diagnoses and can further complicate pre-existing diagnoses, especially if the traumatic event occurs when incarcerated.

Risk Factors McCauley and Brinkley-Rubinstein (2017) identified several risk factors for LGBTQ+ individuals at the intersection of institutionalization and incarceration. These factors include the pathologization of LGBTQ+ and gender nonconforming identities, poverty, minority stress, trauma, victimization, social and family exclusion, mental health issues, limited access to care, and maladaptive coping strategies. Transgender individuals also have higher psychosocial risks, including substance use and sexual risks (McCann & Brown, 2018). Furthermore, internalized and externalized homophobia and transphobia contribute to mental health struggles (Herek et al., 1998). However, many individuals do not seek help due to barriers such as shame, lack of available services, or fear of discrimination

(McCauley & Brinkley-Rubinstein, 2017). Without access to adequate mental health care, LGBTQ+ individuals are more likely to develop maladaptive coping mechanisms, such as engaging in criminal behavior, self-harm, suicidality, or substance abuse. These behaviors then create a self-perpetuating cycle, leaving them increasingly vulnerable to incarceration and institutionalization (McCauley & Brinkley-Rubinstein, 2017).

Trauma People with trauma and whose symptoms meet the criteria for PTSD are a prevalent concern for incarcerated people. Trauma can be a result of a variety of one-time or recurring events, of which many incarcerated people encounter prior to or while incarcerated. One meta-analysis estimated that upwards of 27% of incarcerated men and 38% of incarcerated women have PTSD (Baranyi et al., 2018). Another article looking at prevalence rates for those incarcerated in Illinois compared to the general populace showed a much more grim disparity (Adams et al., 2017). Unfortunately, at the time of this writing, it is challenging to know the prevalence of PTSD for LGBTQ+ people who are incarcerated, as there are no specific studies or meta-analyses with that information.

While we don't have specific rates of PTSD for LGBTQ+ incarcerated, there is research on factors related to trauma and LGBTQ+ incarcerated people, specifically sexual abuse. For example, research has shown that LGBTQ+ individuals who are incarcerated face a heightened risk of sexual abuse and assault during their imprisonment (McCauley & Brinkley-Rubinstein, 2017). More than 67% of LGBTQ+ incarcerated individuals have reported being raped multiple times, which significantly increases their risk of developing physical health issues and PTSD (Neal & Clements, 2010). Additionally, those who are sexually assaulted by fellow incarcerated individuals often sustain physical injuries, while those assaulted by correctional staff report physical abuse in 50% of cases (Neal & Clements, 2010). Moreover, sexual abuse during incarceration frequently leads to the development of avoidance coping strategies and a range of symptoms beyond PTSD, including depression, anger, guilt, disrupted belief systems, and sexual dysfunction (Boeschen et al., 1998). Overall, PTSD has high comorbidity rates with anxiety and depressive disorders, which can further deteriorate overall mental health, especially when someone is at risk of re-traumatization while incarcerated (Qassem et al., 2020).

Impact of Justice System on Mental Health Previous research has shown that any history of involvement with the justice system, from arrest onward, is positively correlated with recent symptoms of depression, anxiety, self-harm, and suicidality among LGBTQ+ youth (Rogers et al., 2022; Trimble, 2019). Research found that 33% of detained LGBTQ+ youth reported having suicidal attempts and 52% of them have active suicidal thoughts (Clark et al., 2022). Since LGBTQ+ youth encounter the justice system at disproportionately higher rates due to various systemic and social factors, and if incarcerated, the unique challenges of being both LGBTQ+ and incarcerated can further exacerbate mental health struggles (Hobaica et al., 2024). After release, these individuals also often face additional challenges such as returning to unsafe homes or communities, which are compounded by other limited resources due to their history of incarceration. These factors, in turn, contribute to heightened risks of recidivism and ongoing mental health concerns (Hobaica et al., 2024).

Relational Challenges

Moreover, research indicates that LGBTQ+ incarcerated individuals often face significant challenges in both family and romantic relationships. Prior research confirms that maintaining family connections benefits the mental health of incarcerated individuals and reduces the likelihood of recidivism (Zamble & Quinsey, 1997). There are various challenges that contribute to an incarcerated individual's ability to maintain good family and romantic relationships.

Youth Relationships Studies show that LGBTQ+ incarcerated youth are at a high risk of homelessness due to family discrimination and rejection. The lack of familial support forces around 40% of LGBTQ+ incarcerated youth into sex work for survival, increasing their vulnerability and exposure to risks, and ultimately contributing to their incarceration (Lydon et al., 2015). While no one person or system can eliminate homophobia and bolster family relationships for LGBTQ+ youth, it is important to know factors that can result in LGBTQ+ youth being incarcerated, and what may increase recidivism rates.

Family Relationships Incarceration affects not only the individual but also their family members, underscoring the need to view incarceration through a systemic. Goldman (2019) found that the incarceration of adult children negatively impacts parental health and strains parent-child relationships. For example, mothers of incarcerated children report experiencing heightened stress, anxiety, depression, and physical ailments (Turney, 2021). When grandchildren are involved, mothers of incarcerated individuals (grandmother) often take on the responsibility of raising them, as well as managing the well-being of other family members or in-laws (Goldman, 2019). The physical absence of the incarcerated individual creates overall strain on the family, especially when family members face their own health challenges.

Unfortunately, family members also often experience shame related to the incarceration, leading to social withdrawal and isolation, exacerbating stress (Sirois, 2020). Financial burdens and coparenting pressures add to these challenges, as family members are left to provide for the household and raise children on their own without the support of their incarcerated loved ones (Tadros et al., 2021; Tadros & Durante, 2022). Other studies have also found that familial conflict is directly linked to higher risks of drug abuse and difficulties during the reentry process (Mowen & Visher, 2015). Incarceration affects the entire family system, and while it is challenging to maintain family relationships while incarcerated, it is critical to strengthen such relationships to help reduce recidivism rates.

Romantic Relationships Conflict between incarcerated individuals and their partners is the second most common factor influencing recidivism (Zamble & Quinsey, 1997). Incarceration has been found to negatively impact the quality of relationships (Hairston, 2003) and contribute to mental health issues and maladaptive coping strategies, such as suicidality and substance use (Carlson & Cervera, 1991). Also, partners of incarcerated individuals often report feelings of shame, anger, and resistance to compromise (Barretti & Beitin, 2010) and are at higher risk for drug and alcohol abuse (Western et al., 2004).

Furthermore, maintaining a quality romantic relationship between incarcerated individuals and their partners is challenging due to several factors, including physical separation, limited opportunities to resolve conflicts, and a lack of both emotional and sexual intimacy (Tadros et al., 2022). Separation from partners results in diminished intimacy, interaction, and quality time (McKay et al., 2018), while the costs of maintaining contact through phone calls and visitation continue to increase (Tadros & Finney, 2018). Incarcerated individuals who suffer from mental health issues often experience increased emotional detachment and isolation, which can further strain relationships (De Claire et al., 2020).

Perhaps unsurprisingly, infidelity, in all forms, occurs at alarmingly high rates—up to 50%—in couples where one partner is incarcerated (Davey-Rothwell et al., 2012). These issues are often rooted in unmet needs for interdependence, intimacy, and sexual reciprocity from the incarcerated partner (Norona et al., 2017). Unfortunately for those who are married prior to or while being incarcerated, Skipper et al. (2020) highlight the high divorce rates among couples separated by incarceration, emphasizing the significant relational barriers posed by imprisonment. This data is important, because much like the family system, the incarcerated individual and their romantic relationship(s) are influential in one's overall physical and mental health. As noted above, if an incarcerated individual's second most common factor influencing recidivism is their romantic relationship, there is a greater need to support the health of such relationships.

Case Study

Similar to the statistics presented, Azul has comorbid diagnoses of Post-Traumatic Stress Disorder (PTSD) and generalized anxiety disorder. Traumatic events stem from houselessness, but also multiple adverse childhood events (ACEs). The symptoms of PTSD are exacerbated by strained peer relationships while incarcerated and brash authoritarian Correctional Officers, who are reminiscent of police officers who have perpetuated harm throughout Azul's life. Relationally, Azul feels they have little support, as they have no romantic partners and are unable to stay in contact with friends and family due to complications of houselessness. While Azul is close with their siblings, their extended family members refuse to facilitate visits or communication, for fear that Azul will negatively influence them.

Recommendations and Treatment

Prison Policies and Recommendations

First and foremost, there is a deep need for governing bodies at the federal and state levels to develop clear, written policies for LGBTQ+ people who are incarcerated. These policies should be written in tandem with mental health and medical professionals and include input from LGBTQ+ people with lived experiences of being incarcerated. Additionally, there are various agencies and associations, such as the National Institute of Corrections, American Correctional Association, and National Commission on Correctional Health Care, who also put forth policies and requirements for best practices and accreditation. These policies should address the key issues and clinical needs as described above. Furthermore, there should be increased programming while incarcerated and supplemental reentry services for a more successful transition out of incarceration and to reduce recidivism rates (Bassichis, 2007).

Gender-Affirming Care

Gender-Affirming care can include a wide variety of interventions and practices to combat gender dysphoria and secondary diagnoses that develop as a result of it, such as depression and anxiety. One of the most prominent organizations addressing transgender health care is the World Professional Association on Transgender Health (WPATH). They have a Standards of Care and an extensive directory of medical and mental health professionals from around the world. It is important to note that adequate care spans medical and mental health treatment options including, but not limited to, hormone replacement therapy (HRT), gender-affirming surgery(ies), and allowing gender-appropriate clothing.

Hormone Replacement Therapy (HRT)

Currently, there is a need for evidence-based policies surrounding access to hormones for gender-affirming transition care while incarcerated. Facilities can ease this burden by allowing transgender and nonbinary individuals to engage in hormone replacement therapy while incarcerated regardless of prior access, diagnoses, or prescriptions. This care should be directed by a medical professional and ensure adequate, continual access to the hormone(s) being prescribed to reduce the risk of misuse or reversal of effects. Policy creation can also be supported by organizations such as WPATH.

Choices for Living Assignments

As noted previously, living assignments are based on differing policies, facilities, and personal circumstances for the incarcerated individual. One of the easiest ways to face this choice with good intent and dignity for those incarcerated is to allow placement of transgender, intersex, and gender nonconforming individuals to their preferred location based on their self-assessment of safety and vulnerability. As of 2024, most prisons and jails still use sex assigned at birth or genitalia as the determining factor. However, some areas have successfully changed that determinant to gender identity, such as in Cook County, IL, Cumberland, ME, Denver, CO, and Washington, D.C. Although these are just a handful of successful instances, it should promote conversation and viable pathways for other locations and institutions to integrate more gender-affirming placement options. Additionally, it is important to note that facilities should avoid confinement or segregation when working with mentally ill incarcerated individuals, as it can increase the risk for self-harm and suicide when segregated or isolated (Abramsky & Fellner, 2003; Lydon et al., 2015).

Mental Health Care

Evidence-based mental health care consistently shows that the best outcomes for treatment are when medication and talk therapy are combined. However, any type of physical or mental health care while incarcerated is often centered on medication, typically due to lack of resources. When talk therapy is offered, individuals often encounter a lack of confidentiality. To improve mental health outcomes during and after incarceration, both types of treatment should be offered consistently.

Specifically, when working with LGBTQ+ clients, it's important to offer culturally competent care to reduce risk of retraumatization and microaggressions (Scott et al., 2019; Sue, 1998). For general case conceptualization, it can be helpful to utilize the minority stress model (Meyer, 2003), which takes into account how LGBTQ+ individuals face proximal (internal) and distal (external) stressors that should both be addressed for adequate treatment (Pantalone et al., 2017). This is similar to utilizing a biopsychosocial model for treatment – addressing the various factors and the impact of their intersections to better treat the concerns and diagnoses as a whole. Of course, it is also critical that all approaches use an intersectional lens, as intersecting marginalized identities bring additional complexity to diagnoses and effective treatment approaches (Bi et al., 2020).

Trauma Treatment

As noted above, PTSD is a common diagnosis occurring across gender identities in the incarcerated setting. Gratefully, there are a multitude of ways that trauma can be addressed or treated, including cognitive behavioral, skills-based, and exposure therapy, including group therapies (Malik et al., 2023). When choosing a treatment modality, there are various factors that play a part in how effective treatment is, including intersectional cultural identities, setting, and resources available.

Cognitive Behavioral Therapy (CBT) and Trauma-Focused CBT (TF-CBT) Cognitive Behavioral Therapy (CBT) continues to be one of the most widely used evidence-based practices in mental health care for a variety of diagnoses. Its foundation focuses on identifying and changing cognitive (thought) distortions to then change behavioral responses. Trauma-Focused CBT was later created to address and process trauma more specifically. Due to its varied applicability and high rates of positive outcomes, it is still one of the highest recommended treatment options, including with incarcerated populations (Tadros et al., 2020; Yoon et al., 2017). It requires few, if any, additional resources beyond those assumed with traditional talk therapy. One study's researchers did acknowledge the benefits of CBT and TF-CBT, but also noted the limitations for treating somatic (bodily) symptoms associated with trauma (Bashir et al., 2023).

Eye Movement Desensitization and Reprocessing (EMDR) EMDR is an evidence-based therapy treatment that was developed in the 1990s and early 2000s focused on processing traumatic events through bilateral stimulation (Shapiro, 2017). The goal of this therapy is to neutralize the negative emotional response to a traumatic event. EMDR is also particularly beneficial for relieving somatic symptoms, such as headaches, stomachaches, and dizziness, that are associated with trauma responses (Gielkens et al., 2022).

A potential drawback of EMDR is that it does require additional training beyond what a traditional educational program offers a mental health professional, and it needs additional resources, such as a light bar or other method of bilateral stimulation. Furthermore, while various research shows EMDR produces promising results for a wide range of individuals, there aren't specific studies that show the efficacy of EMDR for LGBTQ+ individuals who are incarcerated. However, there are some studies that look at the use of EMDR in incarcerated settings.

One qualitative study took place in New Zealand and offered EMDR to individuals diagnosed with PTSD in a long-term forensic care or prison setting (Every-Palmer et al., 2023). An overall theme from participants highlighted how EMDR felt empowering in a very disempowered place. This was particularly true with EMDR therapy in prison, as someone could hold their own thoughts but did not need to articulate them verbally, thereby bypassing limits of confidentiality while incarcerated.

Another study utilized EMDR as a treatment method for individuals diagnosed with PTSD who are incarcerated in the United States (Bashir et al., 2023). The study showed it worked across gender and race, but it is assumed there weren't transgender or nonbinary participants in this study. Overall, the treatment reduced PTSD symptoms. Further research would be beneficial to explore its effectiveness with transgender and nonbinary individuals while incarcerated, but it is still a good foundation for those who are cisgender and not heterosexual.

Group Therapy

Multiple studies also show the benefit of group therapy for incarcerated individuals, both in place of and alongside individual therapy (Davies, 2019; Morgan et al., 2006; Yoon et al., 2017). Group therapy often requires fewer resources being utilized, particularly the time and cost of the mental health professional(s). Additionally, it can give those incarcerated opportunities to learn from each other and find support in one another, especially for those with further marginalized identities or similar experiences (Zielinski et al., 2021). In some situations, it can also help alleviate tensions between those who are incarcerated as well as between correctional staff and those who are incarcerated (Coyne & Fabricatore, 1979). Group therapy in prison settings has been particularly effective for treating concerns such as anger management, general anxiety, and depression (Yoon et al., 2017).

Couples and Family Therapy

In correctional systems, couples and family therapy are not widely indicated compared to individual and group therapy. However, the above challenges describing the impact on families and partners of incarcerated individuals underscore the importance of including families in treatment to improve marital and family satisfaction, strengthen relational bonds, reduce recidivism rates, and increase family cohesion (Bradbury & Bodenmann, 2020; Doss et al., 2022; Gendreau, 1996; Roddy et al., 2020; Shadish & Baldwin, 2003). Marriage and family therapy experts further emphasize systemic and intersectionality viewpoints to examine and mitigate the effects of sociocultural injustice on individual mental health and family relations (Harvey et al., 2021).

A common challenge for incarcerated individuals and their families is communication, and it is key to improving family relationships during incarceration (Song et al., 2018). Family and couples therapy provides a safe space for open dialogue, allowing family members to express their concerns and communicate effectively with the assistance of a professional (Tadros et al., 2023). This process not only helps family members recognize the importance of offering support and love to incarcerated individuals, but it also reduces feelings of detachment (Taylor, 2016). Incarcerated individuals, in turn, experience a sense of belonging and hope as they work with their families (McCann, 1993), such as incarcerated fathers being more inclined to engage in coparenting roles when positive coparenting relationships are in place (Pudasainee-Kapri & Razza, 2015). Additionally, those with a history of incarceration who receive family support are more likely to actively pursue opportunities for financial stability or employment upon release (Mowen & Visher, 2013).

It is also important that couples and family therapies address the disruption of family roles, rules, hierarchy, and structure due to the absence of incarcerated parents (Tadros et al., 2023). In family systems, parents or older family members typically occupy the top of the hierarchy, holding authority. When a family member with authority is incarcerated, family dynamics often become dysfunctional in an attempt to find a new "normal" (Minuchin & Fishman, 1981). Therefore, it is essential to reintegrate these parents, or authority figures back into the family hierarchy during and after incarceration to prevent role confusion and dysfunction.

Furthermore, there are some education programs in correctional systems integrating systemic perspectives for treatment. Parenting education programs aim to enhance parenting attitudes and skills among incarcerated individuals (Palusci et al., 2008). Similarly, an effective intervention called the Prevention and Relationship Enhancement Program, implemented in Oklahoma prisons, focuses on reducing marital distress and divorce by teaching couples relationship skills and principles (Barretti & Beitin, 2010). Such programs exemplify that although family services have traditionally been less available in correctional facilities compared to individual therapy, incorporating couples and family therapy services can play a crucial role in helping them build social connections, reduce the risk of recidivism (Wallace & Wang, 2020), and stabilize families and their communities.

Training for Correctional Officers

Correctional officers (COs) are uniquely poised to provide referrals to mental health care staff since they are with those who are incarcerated on a regular basis and can observe changes in various settings. This advantage means COs could greatly benefit from additional mental health care training to catch concerns and drive referrals sooner, rather than treating all "misbehavior" as deliberate, or feeling responsible for handling mental health issues without support. Such trainings could be created and offered by a variety of organizations with knowledge of the realities of incarceration and needs of LGBTQ+ individuals and their families, such as those mentioned above. Unsurprisingly, COs themselves also deal with high rates of mental illness and burnout, and could also benefit from the trainings for themselves and coworkers (National Institute of Justice, 2023).

Case Study

In an ideal world, Azul would have a variety of resources and choices available to them while incarcerated. They would have access to and an option to start hormones for HRT to reduce gender dysphoria symptoms. They would have a choice for gendered living assignment. Their Correctional Officers would have training on working with LGBTQ+ individuals, including the use of pronouns and intervening and preventing sexual harassment and assault. Azul would also be offered group, individual, and family therapy to treat their mental health diagnoses, such as trauma symptoms from PTSD, increase family connection, and reduce the risk of recidivism upon release.

Limitations

Mental Health Stigma

Across the world, mental health stigma exists, and the U.S. is no exception. Researchers identify three types of stigmas (public, self-, and structural) and how those show up in mental health care (Canada et al., 2022; Singhal, 2024). Over the past three years, there have been general improvements in public stigma related to some mental illness diagnoses, most of which are suspected to be tied to generational shifts (Pescosolido et al., 2021). For incarcerated settings, stigma still exists across all three categories, though most prominently for self- and structural. The results of such stigma often result in barriers to care and refusal for care. Unfortunately, LGBTQ+ individuals face the intersection of multiple types of stigma – for being LGBTQ+, incarcerated, and potentially struggling with mental illness. Of course, stigma cannot be addressed overnight or without considerable effort and education for entire communities.

There is also stigma against family therapy support. Project Greenlight in New York gave incarcerated individuals the option to utilize family therapy as part of the reentry project (Ritter, 2006). This project included cognitive behavioral therapy (CBT) skills, employment assistance, and housing support. However, only about 30% of those eligible and incarcerated volunteered for the family therapy component. While there were various concerns of family member availability, some outrightly denied that there were "family problems" that needed to be addressed.

Lack of Resources

While there are standards for mental health and those incarcerated, prisons are under-resourced in a variety of ways, indicating a lack of commitment to care and upholding such standards (Trimble, 2019). When it comes to offering mental health treatment, a lack of money, time, and trained professionals often means treatment is only offered in group settings (Morgan et al., 1999), and medication is discontinued (Reingle Gonzalez & Connell, 2014). While group therapy is effective, more severe symptoms or those with multiple marginalized identities may be better served by individual therapy. It is estimated that less than 25% of correctional facilities with mental health units offer both group and individual therapy (Cohen et al., 2020).

As discussed above, there are also laws and policies that are created with the intent to protect individuals from sexual assault or issues with living assignments. Specifically, the Prison Rape Elimination Act (PREA) brought much hope for change. However, there are still gaps in implementation follow-through and monitoring (Smith, 2020). Unfortunately, the lack of resources to enforce such laws and policies, such as finances and people advocating for those who are incarcerated, makes it challenging to adequately file a lawsuit for noncompliance.

Lack of Research

For any quality evidence-based practices, there is a need for meaningful and applicable research. There are various studies on parts of this population's identity, but there is a lack of research at the intersection of identities – LGBTQ+, those incarcerated, impact on families and relationships, and mental health needs and treatment. While one can make conjectures about the challenges LGBTQ+ incarcerated people face and what types of treatments and recommendations could be most beneficial, the reality is there is very little research on the intersectional impact of the multiple social identities. To truly serve this population, those supporting incarcerated individuals need more research addressing LGBTQ+ individuals' intersecting identities in this setting (Bauer et al., 2021; Hartwell et al., 2021).

Insufficient Training

In part due to the lack of resources and research, there is also a lack of mental health training for many professionals working with this population. Furthermore, mental health care providers often have little to no exposure to incarcerated settings through their traditional education and typically have as little as one chapter/section on LGBTQ+ care within a broader multicultural counseling course. Often, correctional officers who have the most exposure to incarcerated individuals and interactions with their family members do not receive adequate or appropriate training for handling mental health issues that arise and/or appropriate conduct when working with the LGBTQ+ population that is incarcerated (Darani et al., 2021). While more training would certainly benefit both the professionals and the respective population, there is often a severe lack of time and money available to address this need. Cross-organizational networking such as with local NAMI chapters and those who provide mental health first aid training could help fill the gap with evidence-based baseline training.

Conclusion

This chapter explored key issues, clinical needs, treatment, and systemic policies related to LGBTQ+ adults who are incarcerated, along with the impact on their relationships with partners and families. This population faces a variety of issues that many other incarcerated individuals face, issues non-incarcerated LGBTQ+ people face, and unique challenges for those at the intersection of such identities and circumstances. Unfortunately, there is limited research and resources to address such concerns. Most critically, there is a particular need to better treat and care for transgender and non-binary individuals who are incarcerated, especially with declining sociopolitical attitudes in the U.S. toward this group. Nevertheless, there are still a wide range of opportunities available for professionals in the mental health field and correctional work to learn how to better serve LGBTQ+ people who are incarcerated, and their loved ones, to produce better outcomes for them and their communities at large.

References

Abramsky, S., & Fellner, J. (2003). *Ill equipped: U.S. prisoners and offenders with mental illness.* Human Rights Watch. Retrieved from https://www.hrw.org/report/2003/10/22/ill-equipped/us-prisons-and-offenders-mental-illness

Adams, S., Houston-Kolnik, J., & Reichert, J. (2017, July 25). Trauma-informed and evidence-based practices and programs to address trauma in correctional settings. *Illinois Criminal Justice Information Authority.* Retrieved from https://icjia.illinois.gov/researchhub/articles/trauma-informed-and-evidence-based-practices-and-programs-to-address-trauma-in-correctional-settings

Baranyi, G., Cassidy, M., Fazel, S., Priebe, S., & Mundt, A. P. (2018). Prevalence of posttraumatic stress disorder in prisoners. *Epidemiologic Reviews, 40*(1), 134–145. https://doi.org/10.1093/epirev/mxx015

Barretti, L. M., & Beitin, B. K. (2010). Creating internships in marriage and family therapy: A collaboration between a training program and an offender reentry facility. *Contemporary Family Therapy: An International Journal, 32*, 39–51. https://doi.org/10.1007/s10591-009-9109-3

Bashir, H. A., Wilson, J. F., Ford, J. A., & Hira, N. (2023). Treatment of PTSD and SUD for the incarcerated population with EMDR: A pilot study. *The Journal of Addictions & Offender Counseling, 44*, 132–144. https://doi.org/10.1002/jaoc.12123

Bassichis, D. M. (2007). *It's war in here: A report on the treatment of transgender and intersex people in New York state men's prisons.* New York, NY: The Sylvia Rivera Law Project. https://archive.srlp.org/files/warinhere.pdf

Bauer, G. R., Churchill, S. M., Mahendran, M., Walwyn, C., Lizotte, D., & Villa-Rueda, A. A. (2021). Intersectionality in quantitative research: A systematic review of its emergence and applications of theory and methods. *SSM - Population Health, 14*, 100798. https://doi.org/10.1016/j.ssmph.2021.100798

Bi, S., Vela, M. B., Nathan, A. G., Gunter, K. E., Cook, S. C., López, F. Y., Nocon, R. S., & Chin, M. H. (2020). Teaching intersectionality of sexual orientation, gender identity, and race/ethnicity in a health disparities course. *MedEdPORTAL: The Journal of Teaching and Learning Resources, 16*, 10970. https://doi.org/10.15766/mep_2374-8265.10970

Bradbury, T. N., & Bodenmann, G. (2020). Interventions for couples. *Annual Review of Clinical Psychology, 16*(1), 99–123. https://doi.org/10.1146/annurev-clinpsy-071519-020546

Boeschen, L. E., Sales, B. D., & Koss, M. P. (1998). Rape trauma experts in the courtroom. *Psychology, Public Policy, and Law, 4*(1–2), 414–432. https://doi.org/10.1037/1076-8971.4.1-2.414

Cammett, A. (2009). Queer lockdown: Coming to terms with the ongoing criminalization of LGBTQ communities. *Scholar & Feminist Online*, 613. https://scholars.law.unlv.edu/facpub/613

Canada, K., Barrenger, S., Bohrman, C., Banks, A., & Peketi, P. (2022). Multi-level barriers to prison mental health and physical health care for individuals with mental illnesses. *Frontiers in Psychiatry, 13*, 777124. https://doi.org/10.3389/fpsyt.2022.777124

Carlson, B., & Cervera, N. (1991). Incarceration, coping, and support. *Social Work, 36*, 279–285. https://doi.org/10.1093/sw/36.4.279

Clark, K. A., Harvey, T. D., Hughto, J. M., & Meyer, I. H. (2022). Mental health among sexual and gender minority youth incarcerated in juvenile corrections. *Pediatrics, 150*(6). https://doi.org/10.1542/peds.2022-058158

Cohen, T. R., Mujica, C. A., Gardner, M. E., Hwang, M., & Karmacharya, R. (2020). Mental health units in correctional facilities in the United States. *Harvard Review of Psychiatry, 28*(4), 255–270. https://doi.org/10.1097/HRP.0000000000000267

Coyne, J. C., & Fabricatore, J. M. (1979). Group psychotherapy in a corrections facility: A case study of individual and institutional change. *Professional Psychology, 10*(1), 8–14. https://doi.org/10.1037/0735-7028.10.1.8

Darani, S., Simpson, S., McMaster, R., Wolff, E., Bonato, S., Glancy, G., & Quinn, J. (2021). Mental health training for correctional officers: A systematic review. *BJPsych Open*, *7*(Suppl 1), S18. https://doi.org/10.1192/bjo.2021.104

Davey-Rothwell, M. A., Villarroel, M. A., Grieb, S.D., & Latin, C. A. (2012). Norms, attitudes, and sex behaviors among women with incarcerated main partners. *Journal of Urban Health*, *90*(6), 1151–1165. https://doi.org/10.1007/s11524-012-9749-8

Davies, J. (2019). An examination of individual versus group treatment in correctional settings. In Polaschek, D. L. L., Day, A., & Hollin, C. R. (Eds.), *The Wiley international handbook of correctional psychology* (pp. 575–589). Chichester, UK: Wiley Blackwell. https://doi.org/10.1002/9781119139980.ch36

De Claire, K., Dixon, L., & Larkin, M. (2020). How prisoners and their partners experience the maintenance of their relationship during a prison sentence. *Journal of Community & Applied Social Psychology*, *30*(3), 293–306. https://doi.org/10.1002/casp.244

Dolovich, S. (2011). Strategic segregation in the modern prison. *American Criminal Law Review*, *48*(1), 1–110. Retrieved from https://escholarship.org/uc/item/5tt422r2

Doss, B. D., Roddy, M. K., Wiebe, S. A., & Johnson, S. M. (2022). A review of the research during 2010–2019 on evidence-based treatments for couple relationship distress. *Journal of Marital and Family Therapy*, *48*(1), 283–306. https://doi.org/10.1111/jmft.12552

Every-Palmer, S., Ross, B., Flewett, T., Rutledge, E., Hansby, O., & Bell, E. (2023). Eye movement desensitisation and reprocessing (EMDR) therapy in prison and forensic services: A qualitative study of lived experience. *European Journal of Psychotraumatology*, *14*(2), 2282029. https://doi.org/10.1080/20008066.2023.2282029

Frost, D. M., & Meyer, I. H. (2009). Internalized homophobia and relationship quality among lesbians, gay men, and bisexuals. *Journal of Counseling Psychology*, *56*(1), 97–109. https://doi.org/10.1037/a0012844

Gendreau, P. (1996). The principles of effective intervention with offenders. In Harland A. (Ed.), *Choosing correctional options that work: Defining the demand and evaluating the supply* (pp. 117–130). Thousand Oaks, CA: Sage.

Ghandnoosh, N., & Stammen, E. (2022, June 9). Incarcerated LGBTQ+ adults and youth. *The Sentencing Project*. https://www.sentencingproject.org/reports/incarcerated-lgbtq-adults-and-youth/

Gielkens, E. M. J., Sobczak, S., Rossi, G., & van Alphen, S. P. J. (2022). The feasibility of eye movement desensitization and reprocessing (EMDR) for older adults with posttraumatic stress disorder (PTSD) and comorbid psychiatric and somatic disorders. *Psychological Trauma: Theory, Research, Practice, and Policy*. Advance online publication. https://doi.org/10.1037/tra0001402

Gmelin, J. H., De Vries, Y. A., Baams, L., Aguilar-Gaxiola, S., Alonso, J., Borges, G., Bunting, B., Cardoso, G., Florescu, S., Gureje, O., Karam, E. G., Kawakami, N., Lee, S., Mneimneh, Z., Navarro-Mateu, F., Posada-Villa, J., Rapsey, C., Slade, T., Stagnaro, J. C., Torres, Y., Kessler, R., de Jonge, P., & WHO World Mental Health Survey collaborators. (2022). Increased risks for mental disorders among LGB individuals: Cross-national evidence from the World Mental Health Surveys.

Social Psychiatry and Psychiatric Epidemiology, 57(11), 2319–2332. https://doi.org/10.1007/s00127-022-02320-z

Goldman, A. W. (2019). Linked lives in double jeopardy: Child incarceration and maternal health at midlife. *Journal of Health and Social Behavior, 60*(4), 398–415. https://doi.org/10.1177/0022146519882328

Hairston, C. F. (2003). Prisoners and their families: Parenting issues during incarceration. In Travis, J., & Waul, M. (Eds.), *Prisoners once removed: The impact of incarceration and reentry on children, families, and communities.* Washington, DC: Urban Institute Press.

Harvey, R., Murphy, M. J., Bigner, J. J., & Wetchler, J. L. (2021). *Handbook of LGBTQ-affirmative couple and family therapy* (2nd ed., pp. 259–282). New York, NY: Routledge. https://doi.org/10.4324/9780429274626

Hartwell, E. E., Belous, C. K., Benson, K., Cox, L., Iantaffi, A., McGeorge, C. R., Shipman, D., & Twist, M. L. C. (2021, October). *Clinical guidelines for LGBT-QIA affirming marriage and family therapy.* American Association for Marriage and Family Therapy. Retrieved from https://www.aamft.org/lgbtqiaguidelines

Herek, G. M., Cogan, J. C., Gillis, J. R., & Glunt, E. K. (1998). Correlates of internalized homophobia in a community sample of lesbians and gay men. *Journal of the Gay & Lesbian Medical Association, 2*(1), 17–25.

Hobaica, S., Price, M. N., DeChants, J. P., Davis, C. K., & Nath, R. (2024). Justice involvement and mental health in LGBTQ young people. *Children and Youth Services Review, 160*, 107571. https://doi.org/10.1016/j.childyouth.2024.107571

Hodshire, S. (2023, June 5). *How does HRT change your body during transition?* Healthline. Retrieved from https://www.healthline.com/health/transgender/hrt-effects-on-body

James, S. E., Herman, J. L., Durso, L. E., & Heng-Lehtinen, R. (2024, February). *Early insights: A report of the 2022 U.S. transgender survey.* National Center for Transgender Equality, Washington, D.C.

James, S. E., Herman, J. L., Rankin, S., Keisling, M., Mottet, L., & Anafi, M. (2016). *The report of the 2015 U.S. transgender survey.* National Center for Transgender Equality, Washington, DC.

Khan, M., Ilcisin, M., & Saxton, K. (2017). Multifactorial discrimination as a fundamental cause of mental health inequities. *International Journal for Equity in Health, 16*(1), 43. https://10.1186/s12939-017-0532-z

Lambda Legal. FAQ: Answers to common questions about mistreatment of TGNC incarcerated people. Lambda Legal. https://legacy.lambdalegal.org/know-your-rights/article/trans-in-prison-faq?_gl=1%2A1lban5u%2A_ga%2AMTA2MDI3NjI2LjE3MDcxOTQ0OTk.%2A_ga_290ZG8GMP3%2AMTcwNzE5NDQ5OC4xLjAuMTcwNzE5NDQ5OC42MC4wLjA

Lydon, J., Carrington, K., Low, H., Miller, R., & Yazdy, M. (2015). *Coming out of concrete closets: A report on Black & Pink's National LGBTQ Prisoner Survey.* Black & Pink. https://www.blackandpink.org/wp-content/uploads/Coming-Out-of-Concrete-Closets.pdf

MacInnes, G. A. (2002). Creative politics: Taxes and public goods in a federal system by Glenn beamer. *Journal of Policy Analysis and Management, 21*(3), 518–520. Retrieved from https://search.ebscohost.com/login.aspx?direct=true&AuthTy

pe=ip,sso&db=edsjsr&AN=edsjsr.3325687&site=eds-live&authtype=sso&custid=s8475574

Malik, N., Facer-Irwin, E., Dickson, H., Bird, A., & MacManus, D. (2023). The effectiveness of trauma-focused interventions in prison settings: A systematic review and meta-analysis. *Trauma, Violence & Abuse*, *24*(2), 844–857. https://doi.org/10.1177/15248380211043890

McCann, G. (1993). Relatives' support groups in a special hospital: An evaluation study. *Journal of Advanced Nursing*, *18*(12), 1883–1888. https://doi.org/10.1046/j.1365-2648.1993.18121883.x

McCann, E., & Brown, M. (2018). Vulnerability and psychosocial risk factors regarding people who identify as transgender. A systematic review of the research evidence. *Issues in Mental Health Nursing*, *39*(1), 3–15. https://doi.org/10.1080/01612840.2017.1382623

McCauley, E., & Brinkley-Rubinstein, L. (2017). Institutionalization and incarceration of LGBT individuals. In *Trauma, resilience, and health promotion in LGBT patients: What every healthcare provider should know* (pp. 149–161). https://doi.org/10.1007/978-3-319-54509-7_13

McKay, T., Comfort, M., Grove, L., Bir, A., & Lindquist, C. (2018). Whose punishment, whose crime? Understanding parenting and partnership in a time of mass incarceration. *Journal of Offender Rehabilitation*, *57*(2), 69–82. https://doi.org/10.1080/10509674.2017.1294640

Meyer, I. H. (2003). Prejudice, social stress, and mental health in lesbian, gay, and bisexual populations: Conceptual issues and research evidence. *Psychological Bulletin*, *129*(5), 674–697. https://doi.org/10.1037/0033-2909.129.5.674

Meyer, I. H., Flores, A. R., Stemple, L., Romero, A. P., Wilson, B. D. M., & Herman, J. L. (2017). Incarceration rates and traits of sexual minorities in the United States: National inmate survey, 2011–2012. *American Journal of Public Health (1971)*, *107*(2), 267–273. https://doi.org/10.2105/AJPH.2016.303576

Meyer, I. H., Russell, S. T., Hammack, P. L., Frost, D. M., & Wilson, B. D. M. (2021). Minority stress, distress, and suicide attempts in three cohorts of sexual minority adults: A U.S. probability sample. *PloS One*, *16*(3), e0246827–e0246827. https://doi.org/10.1371/journal.pone.0246827

Minuchin, S., & Fishman, H. C. (1981). *Family therapy techniques.* Cambridge, MA: Harvard University Press.

Morgan, R. D., Kroner, D. G., & Mills, J. F. (2006). Group psychotherapy in prison: Facilitating change inside the walls. *Journal of Contemporary Psychotherapy: On the Cutting Edge of Modern Developments in Psychotherapy*, *36*(3), 137–144. https://doi.org/10.1007/BF02729057

Morgan, R. D., Winterowd, C. L., & Ferrell, S. W. (1999). A national survey of group psychotherapy services in correctional facilities. *Professional Psychology: Research and Practice*, *30*(6), 600–606. https://doi.org/10.1037/0735-7028.30.6.600

Mowen, T. J., & Visher, C. A. (2015). Drug use and crime after incarceration: The role of family support and family conflict. *Justice Quarterly*, *32*(2), 337–359. https://doi.org/10.1080/07418825.2013.771207

National Inmate Survey. (2012). *National Inmate Survey (NIS)*. https://bjs.ojp.gov/data-collection/national-inmate-survey-nis

National Institute of Justice. (2023, December 1). Research on the mounting problem of correctional officer stress. *National Institute of Justice*. Retrieved from https://nij.ojp.gov/topics/articles/research-mounting-problem-correctional-officer-stress

National PREA Resource Center. (n.d.). Prison Rape Elimination Act. *National PREA Resource Center*. Retrieved from https://www.prearesourcecenter.org/about/prison-rape-elimination-act

Neal, T. M. S., & Clements, C. B. (2010). Prison rape and psychological sequelae: A call for research. *Psychology, Public Policy, and Law*, *16*(3), 284–299. https://doi.org/10.1037/a0019448

Norona, J. C., Olmstead, S. B., & Welsh, D. P. (2018). Betrayals in emerging adulthood: A developmental perspective of infidelity. *The Journal of Sex Research*, *55*(1), 84–98. https://doi.org/10.1080/00224499.2017.1342757

Palusci, V. J., Crum, P., Bliss, R., & Bavolek, S. J. (2008). Changes in parenting attitudes and knowledge among inmates and other at risk populations after a family nurturing program. *Children and Youth Services Review*, *30*, 79–89. https://doi.org/10.1016/j.childyouth.2007.06.006

Pantalone, D. W., Valentine, S. E., & Shipherd, J. C. (2017). Working with survivors of trauma in the sexual minority and transgender and gender nonconforming populations. In DeBord, K. A., Fischer, A. R., Bieschke, K. J. & Perez, R. M. (Eds.), *Handbook of sexual orientation and gender diversity in counseling and psychotherapy* (pp. 183–211). Washington, DC: American Psychological Association. https://doi.org/10.1037/15959-008

Pescosolido, B. A., Halpern-Manners, A., Luo, L., & Perry, B. (2021). Trends in public of mental illness in the US, 1996–2018. *JAMA Network Open*, *4*(12), e2140202. https://doi.org/10.1001/jamanetworkopen.2021.40202

Pudasainee-Kapri, S., & Razza, R. A. (2015). Associations among supportive coparenting, father engagement and attachment: The role of race/ethnicity. *Journal of Child and Family Studies*, *24*(12), 3793–3804. https://doi.org/10.1007/s10826-015-0187-6

Qassem, T., Aly-ElGabry, D., Alzarouni, A., Abdel-Aziz, K., & Arnone, D. (2021). Psychiatric co-morbidities in post-traumatic stress disorder: Detailed findings from the adult psychiatric morbidity survey in the English population. *The Psychiatric Quarterly*, *92*(1), 321–330. https://doi.org/10.1007/s11126-020-09797-4

Reingle Gonzalez, J. M., & Connell, N. M. (2014). Mental health of prisoners: Identifying barriers to mental health treatment and medication continuity. *American Journal of Public Health*, *104*(12), 2328–2333. https://doi.org/10.2105/AJPH.2014.302043

Ritter, N. (2006). No shortcuts to successful reentry: The failings of project greenlight. *Corrections Today*, *68*(7), 94–95, 97. Retrieved from https://ezproxy.messiah.edu/login?url=https://www.proquest.com/trade-journals/no-shortcuts-successful-reentry-failings-project/docview/215695659/se-2

Roddy, M. K., Walsh, L. M., Rothman, K., Hatch, S. G., & Doss, B. D. (2020). Meta-analysis of couple therapy: Effects across outcomes, designs, timeframes, and other moderators. *Journal of Consulting and Clinical Psychology*, *88*(7), 583–596. https://doi.org/10.1037/ccp0000514

Rogers, E. M., Krajewski, A. T., & Shuster, S. M. (2022). The disproportionate mental health burden among incarcerated transgender and gender diverse people. *Journal of Correctional Health Care, 29*(1), 39–46. https://doi.org/10.1089/jchc.21.10.0109

Scott, S. B., Whitton, S. W., & Buzzella, B. A. (2019). Providing relationship interventions to same-sex couples: Clinical considerations, program adaptations, and continuing education. *Cognitive and Behavioral Practice, 26*(2), 270–284. https://doi.org/10.1016/j.cbpra.2018.03.004

Shapiro, F. (2017). *Eye movement desensitization and reprocessing (EMDR) therapy: Basic principles, protocols, and procedures.* New York, NY: Guilford Publications.

Shadish, W. R., & Baldwin, S. A. (2003). Meta-analysis of MFT interventions. *Journal of Marital and Family Therapy, 29*(4), 547–570. https://doi.org/10.1111/j.1752-0606.2003.tb01694.x

Singhal, N. (2024, March). *Stigma, prejudice and discrimination against people with mental illness.* American Psychiatric Association. Retrieved from https://www.psychiatry.org/patients-families/stigma-and-discrimination

Sirois, C. (2020). The strain of sons' incarceration on mothers' health. *Social Science & Medicine (1982), 264,* 113264–113264. https://doi.org/10.1016/j.socscimed.2020.113264

Skipper, A. D., Bates, D. S., Blizard, Z. D., & Moye, R. G. (2020). Charged with instability: Are paternal arrests and criminal charges enough to shake the marital stability of American couples? *Journal of Family Issues, 41*(12), 2423–2447. https://doi.org/10.1177/0192513x20942813

Smith, H. P. (2020). Evaluating the implementation of the Prison Rape Elimination Act (PREA): A "Lessons Learned" approach. *Evaluation and Program Planning, 83,* 101855. https://doi.org/10.1016/j.evalprogplan.2020.101855

Song, H., Woo, Y., Lee, H. D., & Cochran, J. K. (2018). The dynamics of intra-family relationships during incarceration and the implications for children of incarcerated parents. *International Journal of Offender Therapy and Comparative Criminology, 62,* 3775–3796. https://doi.org/10.1177/0306624X18755481

Srivastava, A., Prost, S. G., & Williams, S. M. (2023). Mental health among lesbian, gay, bisexual and other non-heterosexual adults in United States Prisons. *Current Psychology: A Journal for Diverse Perspectives on Diverse Psychological Issues, 42*(31), 27709–27718. https://doi.org/10.1007/s12144-022-03777-6

Sue, S. (1998). In search of cultural competence in psychotherapy and counseling. *American Psychologist, 53*(4), 440–448. https://doi.org/10.1037/0003-066X.53.4.440

Taylor, C. J. (2016). The family's role in the reintegration of formerly incarcerated individuals: The direct effects of emotional support. *The Prison Journal, 96*(3), 331–354. https://doi.org/10.1177/0032885516635085

Tadros, E., & Durante, K. A. (2022). Coparenting, negative educational outcomes, and familial instability in justice-involved families. *International Journal of Offender Therapy and Comparative Criminology, 66,* 267–287. https://doi.org/10.1177/0306624X211013740

Tadros, E., Fanning, K., Jensen, S., & Poehlmann-Tynan, J. (2021). Coparenting and mental health in families with jailed parents. *International Journal of Environmental Research and Public Health, 18*(16), 8705. https://doi.org/10.3390/ijerph18168705

Tadros, E., & Finney, N. (2018). Structural family therapy with incarcerated families: A clinical case study. *The Family Journal*, 26, 253–261. https://doi.org/10.1177/0306624X18821825

Tadros, E., Hutcherson, R., & Aguirre, N. (2023). How is family therapy discussed in the literature on incarceration?: A systematic review. *The American Journal of Family Therapy*, *51*(5), 673–691. https://doi.org/10.1080/01926187.2022.2031343

Tadros, E., Presley, S., & Gomez, E. (2022). "Not for the Weak": The lived experience of women in romantic relationships with incarcerated individuals. *Crime & Delinquency*, *68*(12), 2274–2297. https://doi.org/10.1177/00111287221077657

Tadros, E., Ribera, E., Campbell, O., Kish, H., & Ogden, T. (2020). A call for mental health treatment in incarcerated settings with transgender individuals. *American Journal of Family Therapy*, *48*(5), 495–508. https://doi-org.ezproxy.messiah.edu/10.1080/01926187.2020.1761273

Trimble, P. E. (2019). Ignored LGBTQ prisoners: Discrimination, rehabilitation, and mental health services during incarceration. *LGBTQ Policy Journal*, *9*, 31–37.

Turney, K. (2021). Family Member incarceration and mental health: Results from a nationally representative survey. *SSM - Mental Health*, *1*, 100002. https://doi.org/10.1016/j.ssmmh.2021.100002

Wallace, D., & Wang, X. (2020). Does in-prison physical and mental health impact recidivism? *SSM-Population Health*, *11*, 100569. https://doi.org/10.1016/j.ssmph.2020.100569

Western, B., Lopoo, L. M., & McLanahan, S. (2004). Incarceration and the bonds among parents in fragile families. In Patillo, M., Weiman, D., & Western, B. (Eds.), *Imprisoning America: The social effects of mass incarceration* (pp. 21–45). New York: Russell Sage Foundation.

White Hughto, J. M., Clark, K. A., Altice, F. L., Reisner, S. L., Kershaw, T. S., & Pachankis, J. E. (2018). Creating, reinforcing, and resisting the gender binary: A qualitative study of transgender women's healthcare experiences in sex-segregated jails and prisons. *International Journal of Prisoner Health*, *14*(2), 69–88. https://doi.org/10.1108/IJPH-02-2017-0011

Yoon, I. A., Slade, K., & Fazel, S. (2017). Outcomes of psychological therapies for prisoners with mental health problems: A systematic review and meta-analysis. *Journal of Consulting and Clinical Psychology*, *85*(8), 783–802. https://doi.org/10.1037/ccp0000214

Zamble, E., & Quinsey, V. (1997). *Cambridge studies in criminology. The criminal recidivism process.* Cambridge: Cambridge University Press.

Zielinski, M. J., Karlsson, M. E., & Bridges, A. J. (2021). "I'm not alone, my story matters": Incarcerated women's perspectives on the impact and acceptability of group psychotherapy involving imaginal exposure to sexual assault memories. *Health & Justice*, *9*(25). Retrieved from https://doi.org/10.1186/s40352-021-00148-4

Chapter 7

The U.S. Correctional System

Punitive or Rehabilitative?

Jeffrey Shewell and Eman Tadros

In 1757, despite being a time at which the ideals of the European Enlightenment were at their apex, when discourse around the dignity and rights of man was widespread, and during the advent of Western democratic movements, French newspapers described, in grisly and unsettling detail, the public torture and subsequent execution, abhorrent in nature and unfathomable to a modern-day audience, and an act in complete defiance of the philosophical and socio-political zeitgeist of the time, of Robert-François Damiens, a man convicted of the attempted assassination of King Louis XIV, then King of France. As if the eye of the on-looking public was insufficient enough to dehumanize the condemned man, a recounting and proliferation of his slaughter set to print, available to the French public, and now accessible to the modern reader abroad more than two and a half centuries later, further served to punish, humiliate, and eternalize the torturous demise of the would-be regicide (Foucault, 1975)

Not more than two decades passed before many of the "founding fathers" of the United States, Thomas Jefferson and Benjamin Franklin among them, argued that corporal punishment in the pursuit of legal justice – upon which the public often gazed with spectacle – was "inherently despotic and immoral in nature"; viewed by them to be "native weapons of kings" (McLennan, 2008, p. 19). The birth of a newly founded democratic republic, fixated on liberty and the "unalienable rights" of the individual, "endowed by their creator," would simultaneously see the death of a justice system understood by the "founders" of the nation as one both cruel and inhumane. But while it could be argued that this perspective was emblematic of a more enlightened view of criminal justice–a view more moral, more humane–held by a people wishing to break free from the monarchical traditions of the tyrannical autocrats of 18th century Western Europe, and although in some ways it was, the decision to shift away from corporal and capital punishment and toward incarceration was also a pragmatic one. A pragmatic decision, with political and economic benefits, setting a precedent which would influence

DOI: 10.4324/9781003542940-7

the function and mechanics of the United States prison apparatus, up to and into the 21st century. Benjamin Rush, physician, "founding father" of the United States, and signatory to the U.S. Declaration of Independence, was a leading figure in the post-revolutionary American movement for penal reform. Rush was a vocal critic of the death penalty, who also argued that all forms of corporal punishment, especially enacted before a public audience, was not only immoral and inhumane, but also challenged the legitimacy of the governing bodies of the new republic, as well as counterproductive to meeting the economic and social needs of an emerging nation still in its infancy (Goodman, 1934).

Rush believed that a law-abiding and morally upright citizenry would support and strengthen the stability of a newly founded democratic state. Punishment, through imprisonment, centered on a philosophy intent on the rehabilitation of criminally minded individuals, as opposed to justice exercised through capital or other forms of corporal punishment, increased the breadth of such citizenry, increasing the strength of the new republic, in ways that punishment merely intent on removing the criminal element from society never could (Goodman, 1934). The methods by which this criminal element would apparently be rehabilitated, rather than eliminated, and the rationale behind such methods, are to be discussed. However, desirable economic benefits, an anticipated outcome of the shift away from corporal and capital punishment and toward incarceration, which equally served as a contributing factor to such reform, and which permeates the American incarceration system to this day.

Prison System: Punitive or Rehab

To understand the ways that the very architecture of prisons is designed to isolate individuals informs how to evaluate the impacts that this confinement has on people in prison, especially considering the large numbers of those in confinement. Through the design of the Panopticon prison in the 1700s, incarcerated individuals were effectively isolated in single cells that prohibited them from being able to see their peers (Davis, 2003). Simultaneously, in this model, prison staff have full visibility of each prison cell, which effectively deprives incarcerated individuals of social interactions while instilling a presence of constant surveillance (Davis, 2003). Other prison reformers advocated for similar prison models that promoted isolation in their architecture throughout the 18th and 19th centuries (Davis, 2003). Much of the impetus for isolating conditions in prisons were centered around the goals of reform, in the way that that incarcerated individuals' would be afforded the opportunity to be in solitude and read the bible, which was reminiscent of a monastic life (Davis, 2003).

The first panopticon prison in America was built in Philadelphia in 1826 as the Western State Penitentiary (Davis, 2003). Eventually, prisons with single cells became the prominent choice for prison construction and solitary confinement continued despite notable concerns (Davis, 2003). In 1842, Charles Dickens had described solitary confinement as being a cruel form of punishment (Davis, 2003). Notably, in 1890, the Supreme Court had acknowledged the damages associated with the use of solitary confinement (Grassian, 2006). Despite these significant recognitions of the dangers of solitary confinement as it relates to psychiatric health, isolating prison models and practices have remained common into the 21st century. As of the early 2000s, there were at least 60 super maximum prison facilities in America that largely keep incarcerated individuals locked down and isolated for 23 hours each day of the week (Davis, 2003). Pointing to this history of prison design emphasizes the ways that current prison models and practices are outdated, and do not align with what we now know about the pervasive, harmful nature of solitary confinement and what it means to reform and rehabilitate. Tracing the current prison model and confinement practices in America back to religion as a function of reform and forced monasticism raises momentous questions about the persistence of solitary confinement and prison designs, especially considering the ongoing concerns and evidence of its effects.

The early prison system, starting with revolutionary America, approached the prison like a monastery, very religious in nature. In addition to the historic use of incarceration and isolation with the intention to reform individuals, confinement has also been used to detach those with mental illness from society. During America's colonial period, those with mental illnesses were imprisoned alongside criminals under the belief that their psychiatric conditions were attributed to evil (Grassian, 2006). There is an alarming connection between current incarceration trends after the deinstitutionalization movement and the makeup of colonial prisons. The deinstitutionalization movement that began in the United States in the 1950s sought to provide mental health care outside of institutions in community settings instead (Onah, 2018). Gaps in mental health care and the lack of adequate community treatment paths have left many without treatment, especially upon release from institutions in the 1980s (Onah, 2018). The resulting effects of Medicaid exclusions that began in 1965, which limited treatment eligibility and options for mentally ill patients, continue to this day (Onah, 2018).

The Institutions for Mental Disorder (IMD) exclusions in the Medicaid Act further limited eligibility for institutional mental health care, as well as capacities in state-run hospitals for psychiatric care. Between 1955 and 2013, the number of psychiatric beds in state-run hospitals decreased from 500,000 to 35,000 (Onah, 2018). This timeline overlaps with the proliferation of prisons in the United States and a dramatic rise in the prison population (Davis, 2003). This substantial rise in the prison population between 1980 and 2009 notably did not correlate with higher crime rates, but rather "tough on crime" sentiments that accompanied more policing and harsher sentencing (Shjarback & Young, 2017). With further restrictions and barriers to institutional mental health care, those with severe mental illnesses became vulnerable to homelessness, and thus more vulnerable to interactions with police and incarceration (Onah, 2018). Approximately 33% of homeless people are believed to be mentally ill and are often incarcerated for low-level offenses such as trespassing, drug use, public intoxication, public urination, disorderly conduct, or petty theft (Onah, 2018). Understanding the context behind ways that patients are funneled into the prison system can outline care needs and highlight the demand for treatment in incarceration settings, as well as less harmful prison practices and prison alternatives.

Family members also need to be educated on their role in the re-assimilation of formerly incarcerated individuals and the need for their involvement to decrease the likelihood of re-offense. Some family members may alienate the incarcerated person, "disown" them. The focus needs to be not only on the incarcerated individual but on the family member as well. If familial support is necessary to prevent re-offense, then the family members themselves are recommended to attempt to understand and support the incarcerated individual. As therapists, we can promote relationships and family connections all we want to the post-release individual, but if there's no family there to embrace them, what good does it do? Incarcerated individuals are frequently ostracized by their family members. How do we decrease that ostracization?

"Rehabilitation" through Incarceration in Its Infancy – A Repeat Cycle

There are consequences to the ostracization caused by incarceration. Dr. Gabor Mate studies Attention-Deficit/Hyperactivity Disorder (ADHD) and argues in his *Scattered*, that the "attention-deficit" in ADHD is not referring to an inability to "pay attention," but in fact, *a deficit of attention being paid*, to the afflicted child (Mate, 1999, p. 19). This turns on its head the negative connotations associated with the phrase, "attention seeking behavior" (Mate, 1999, p. 22). Kids act out because they're being deprived of attention! So, what do we typically do to address their "acting out"? We put them in time-out, send them to their room, withhold things from them, ultimately depriving them even more of the attention that they so desperately need in order to feel safe and whole and loved! The very deprivation that has contributed to their "misbehavior" in the first place. Our punishment fuels the very "crime" we're seeking to punish.

"Rehabilitation" through Incarceration Today

Recent literature explores a lack of support and services within the correctional system, how many of the same approaches from the early days are still present today and the same shortcomings are just as present as a result. Make it evident that the current system does little in the way of rehabilitating those incarcerated. Effectively, individuals living with severe mental illnesses who are incarcerated instead of treated are ostracized from society in a way that is ominously similar to incarcerated individuals in Colonial America. In both cases, the isolation and ostracization is in many ways attributed to their conditions. These connections further express the ways that additional characteristics of the criminal justice system are dated and do not properly respond to the needs of those requiring treatment or reflect a current understanding of psychiatric health needs. While some efforts such as mental health and drug courts currently exist to provide alternatives to incarceration, their establishment is nowhere near systematic (American Psychological Association [APA], 2014). These treatment deficits and susceptibility to incarceration further stresses needs for alternatives to incarceration and also speak to the problematic nature of solitary confinement.

Economic Benefits of a Highly Incarcerated State

While the architects of the United States, among them Benjamin Rush and Thomas Jefferson, sought the construction of a form of government starkly contrasted with the monarchies of the "old world," pursuing such aims in part through a reformation of the treatment of convicted criminals, such figures also remained keenly aware of the tangible gains, namely economic in nature, to be had by such reforms. In contemporary times, when the notion of a privately-run, for-profit incarceration facility is no longer a thing of suspicion or speculation, but a matter of reality and a part of the American experience, it is pertinent to trace such an economic arrangement back to its infancy, back to a time when the United States was itself in its own infancy as well.

Although Benjamin Rush convincingly argued for the abolition of the death penalty, as well as of other forms of corporal punishment, outlining the detriment that such forms of retribution could cause society, he simultaneously argued that, not only could such penal reform eliminate the burden bore on social welfare caused by traditional forms of criminal justice, but such reform could benefit society in a net-positive way as well. Goodman et. al. identifies the intentions behind Rush's passionate call for reform as being not one exclusively devoted to the reformation of the individual but also one intent on "generating revenue for the state" (Goodman, 1934, p.23). Although corporal punishment could be argued to serve as a deterrent against crime, and capital punishment (also a deterrent) as a means to completely eliminate criminal actors from society, penal institutions could do the same, while also taking advantage of the cheap labor incarcerated individuals could provide, the only cost associated with such arrangement being the necessary provisions – food, shelter, minimal health care – to keep them alive and physically healthy enough to work.

Sharing an attitude similar to that of Rush, Thomas Jefferson argued in his 1789 *A Bill for Proportioning Crimes and Punishments Heretofore Capital*, that the penitentiary approach offered the potential for the reformation of criminals, rather than simply their elimination from society, while also providing the state with an opportunity for incarcerated individuals to be "rendered useful in various labors for the public," an opportunity lost if the individual is executed or simply dealt a corporal punishment and subsequently released (Jefferson, 1779, p. 1). Outlining proposed punishments for a variety of crimes, for those that did not result in the physical harm of another person, Jefferson's bill relies almost exclusively on a sentencing to "hard labor in the public works" for varied durations of time (Jefferson, 1779, p. 2).

To detractors who may have argued that such punishment was insufficiently punitive, those in favor of reform noted that a deprivation of "liberty," an enlightenment ideal highly treasured at the time of the American Revolution, was comparable to traditional judicial penalties in terms of severity (McLennan, 2009). Criminal justice reform within the newly founded United States therefore would become more "humane" while remaining sufficiently punitive for the committed crime, while producing the socio-economic benefit of providing a new source of labor for the country. The economic benefits of a population of incarcerated individuals would evolve and take different forms, with new beneficiaries emerging, over the centuries to come, however, the potentially lucrative nature of incarceration has remained a constant in the US prison system up to the present and its evolution will be explored later in this chapter.

Privatization

A part of the incarceration costs may be motivated by the burgeoning privatization of the prison system. Private prisons hold 8% of all American incarcerated; however, a large portion of the justice system has also been privatized including fine collection, court operations, community-based services and treatment, probation supervision, parole supervision, residential facility operations, and jail operations (Lindsey et al., 2016). This could lead to negative outcomes for incarcerated parental individuals as court-associated debt and privatized net widening could lead to financial insecurity, and thus higher recidivism rates. It is important to note that the financial incentive may motivate private parole and court systems to target the collection of fines forgoing a focus on rehabilitation and transition assistance to the formerly incarcerated; this potential challenge is present in both private and public systems as the focus on rehabilitation strays away, leading to post-incarceration impacts in employment, housing, and in empowering individuals from staying free from future charges (Human Rights Watch, 2014).

It is also important to consider the privatization impact on incarcerated parents as it could significantly change outcomes such as recidivism rates, addiction treatments, parole, and transition into the home. Private-run prisons and services may open the door for corruptive practices and redistribution of programs and services for budgetary concerns; business models largely have monetary concerns rather than humanitarian. The privatization element is multilayered, as even some state-run prisons have many aspects that are privatized in the form of contracts to perform drug treatment, health care, and education (Camp & Gaes, 2001)

Studies are sparse into the impact of private and government-run corrections facilities and programs, the ones that do exist omit key services and programs leading to only approximate conclusions on the debate. (Lindsey et al., 2016). A key criticism is that privatization leads to more people getting wrapped up in the criminal justice system leading to more restrictive social control due the financial incentive of having an extensive correctional population (Blomberg et al., 2011).

In Angela Davis' 2003 book, *Are Prisons Obsolete,* she presents challenges to the overall use of incarceration and asserts the possibility of a society with alternative institutions, while also highlighting the structural inequalities present surrounding mass incarceration. The parts of this book that remain relevant to the purpose of this piece relate to the history behind prison design, as well as their intended functions. Davis (2003) points to utilitarian philosopher, Jeremy Bentham, who had conceptualized the panopticon prison, which incorporated a single cell design that isolated the views of incarcerated individuals. The function of this design aligned with the utilitarian principle of maximizing value, and the belief that this isolation would lead to reform and rehabilitation (Davis, 2003).

Other early prisons followed suit with isolating conditions by design that were built to encourage incarcerated individuals to live almost monastically and read the bible as a path to rehabilitation (Davis, 2003). The proliferation of prisons in America and the constructions of supermax facilities maintain elements of this design in the present day (Davis, 2003). Knowing the severe damage that solitary confinement and isolation can have on an individual, there can especially be arguments made against this practice in prison on the sole basis that it does not align with principles of reform or rehabilitation, seeing as it is detrimental to a person. The history of isolation in incarceration facilities should also inform approaches to mental health assessments and treatment, for the reason that given the isolating design, it is possible for all incarcerated individuals to be impacted by the effects of such an environment

How Do We Stop Lying to Ourselves?

It appears that MFTs can be super helpful in this endeavor. If any supporter of the current system of incarceration in the United States is to claim that it is rehabilitative in nature, then they are likely lying. In order to prove themselves neither, they must take up the cause for the reform of the US incarceration system by making the following changes: Go over suggested reforms that would transform the prison system from one of punishment to one of rehabilitation. MFTs can promote transparency about incarceration (Tadros et al., 2023). Correctional facilities should provide information about the booking and incarceration process, as well as the potential mental and emotional impacts of incarceration (Tadros et al., 2021).

Barriers to MFT

Although families should receive government assistance, many are denied support under the Personal Responsibility and Work Opportunity Reconciliation Act (PRWORA) (Morgan et al., 2022). This denial reflects deep-seated societal marginalization (Morgan et al., 2022). The exclusion of impartial families from assistance is a form of systemic marginalization akin to incarceration (Morgan et al., 2022). Due to PRWORA's restrictions on assistance for those with criminal misconduct, families are more likely to face continued scrutiny and stigmatization (Morgan et al., 2022). To promote greater inclusion, policies that recognize diverse family structures while ensuring proper screening and security should be considered (Swanson et al., 2013). Wherever possible, restoring, strengthening, and preserving connections with children and family members may enhance the institution's and, ultimately, the community reintegration's potential benefits. However, maintaining contact with an incarcerated loved one is challenging due to the long distances required for in-person visits and the high cost of phone calls.

Tough on Crime and Mass Incarceration

To properly contextualize an analysis of the impacts of incarceration and solitary confinement, as well as what the clinical implications are, it is necessary to understand more of the recent nature of how incarceration has operated in America. Shjarback and Young (2017) focus on widespread tough on crime attitudes that dominated the political landscape, influenced policy, and widespread attitudes. It is also important to use this information to align with a rise in incarceration after deinstitutionalization movements took hold. This information can be used to know more about the prison population, especially with consideration to Medicaid exclusions that can make more people vulnerable to interactions with law enforcement, and thus incarceration (Onah, 2018). This allows for the identification of ways that vulnerable groups were more likely to be funneled into incarceration, rather than to receive treatment.

Aside from the gaps and barriers to treatment that exist in the public sphere, additional barriers to treatment also exist within incarceration facilities (APA, 2014). These findings display a systemic mishandling of those suffering from mental health conditions in our society. This further informs clinical implications through the ways that the prison population is at an especial risk for their placement in environments designed to isolate and deprive, while simultaneously continuing the cycle of treatment barriers they experienced prior to incarceration.

The wealth of information accomplished by social scientists and research effectively displays the criminal justice system straying from rehabilitation into punitive measures that stretch beyond the walls of imprisonment in the form of oppressive barriers to the previously incarcerated. Social programs have been ineffective at stemming the tide of incarcerated-related negative outcomes to the imprisoned and their familial community. What is needed is a built-in focus on the rehabilitation in criminal justice that follows into post-incarceration and a readjustment in draconian criminal policies that serve as barriers to incarcerated individuals transition back into the family and society. New forms of privatization in prison systems and programs fail to significantly improve incarcerated individuals' outcomes and in many cases were linked to detrimental outcomes.

The Risks and Impacts of Solitary Confinement

Correctional facilities in America require a unique set of needs for treatment in response to the makeup of its prison population and widespread use of isolation. Within incarceration facilities in America, there are high rates of mental illness and those with a history of substance abuse (APA, 2014). The lack of abundant mental health and drug courts for incarceration alternatives, deficits in mental health care and eligibility, as well as the susceptibility to incarceration for vulnerable groups, all lend context to this detail about the prison population. Clinicians who treat people who are or were incarcerated, must be aware of the prevalence of mental illness and substance abuse within incarceration settings. An estimated 50% of people in prison struggle with substance abuse, while approximately 56% of people in state prison are believed to have a mental illness (Smith, 2013). Conditions of prisons and the prevalence of various forms of violence are also risk factors that impact the mental health of a person who has been incarcerated. 9.6% of incarcerated individuals are sexually abused by either another incarcerated individual, or staff member at the prison and about 10% are injured in a fight (Smith, 2013). Other inherent conditions of prison, such as the use of solitary confinement, tense environment, lack of privacy, noisy conditions, poor diet, and the removal from family and community also act as factors that can impact the mental health of an incarcerated individual (Smith, 2013). This makes it evident that many people who are incarcerated are likely to experience specific traumatic events and ongoing discomfort while in prison that impacts their mental health, which should inform a clinician or mental health professional's approach to treatment and also raise concerns over the risks of solitary confinement.

The impact on family members of having a loved one incarcerated is so significant, with such wide-reaching ripples, that some form of family therapy is almost critical for the well-being of the family. The state, prisons, etc., would never recommend it, but independent of post-release or re-entry, there's a need for therapeutic intervention targeted at families with incarcerated loved ones at the moment of incarceration and then indefinitely. So, if the state won't suggest it, there's almost a need to create clinics outside the locations of prison complexes. Or any city with an adjacent prison. A clinic that offers therapy/social work that accepts ALL insurances, specifically low-income, state-funded insurances, and advertises itself as a resource for the families of incarcerated individuals.

Mental health professionals should also be aware of how common the use of solitary confinement is, and what this means for treating, assessing, and diagnosing patients. While rates of solitary confinement are high, many who are never placed in solitary confinement still reside within an environment that has had a historical architecture that creates conditions that are isolating and significantly deprive them of typical sensory experiences. Similarities exist with the symptoms and impacts of sensory deprivation and solitary confinement (Grassian, 2006). For this reason, it is crucial to consider the potential for all people in prison to be impacted in this way, given the dominant prison design models. It's especially notable how even more incarcerated individuals are likely to have experienced solitary confinement due to mitigation efforts in response to the high rates of COVID-19 in prisons. Solitary confinement has been noted to exacerbate existing mental health conditions, as well as result in different assortments of symptoms (Grassian, 2006). To present the common nature of such effects, 50% of California incarcerated individuals in solitary confinement had reported common symptoms that accompany solitary confinement, which include hypersensitivity to light and noise, anxiety, hallucinations, depression, obsessive thoughts, and paranoia (Reiter et al., 2020). Mental health professionals working with incarcerated or formerly incarcerated patients should note the overlaps between the symptoms that solitary confinement produces, while also being aware of the fact that certain combinations of these symptoms do not always align with a particular mental illness (Grassian, 2006). Encountering this population in treatment should involve consideration of these effects, and those overlapping symptoms, such as anxiety, could be connected with the consequences of isolation.

In addition to an awareness of the impacts of solitary confinement, proper measures to assess and identify these impacts are necessary. These combinations of symptoms associated with isolation do not typically align with existing mental health assessment tools (Reiter et al., 2020). This poses further challenges to mental health professionals, especially considering that those with mental illnesses are more likely to be placed in solitary confinement due to a decreased ability to abide by prison rules (Grassian, 2006). Through re-interviewing people who were placed in solitary confinement and experienced psychological distress as a result, it has been found that these symptoms continue, and can often be permanent (Reiter et al., 2020). This presents further difficulty with adjusting to not only the general prison population after release from solitary confinement, but with life outside of prison upon release, with solitary confinement and sensory deprivation resulting in persisting post-traumatic stress disorder (PTSD), adjustment issues, difficulty functioning in social settings, anxiety, paranoia, hallucinations, depression, and sensory sensitivities (Grassian, 2006). Mental health professionals should be prepared to consider and identify the effects of sensory deprivation in all people who are or have been incarcerated and especially within those who have been placed in solitary confinement. This is especially since traditional assessment tools may not be reliable in identifying these effects, and also since there may be hesitance on behalf of patients to report these symptoms as a self-protection effort, which aligns with prison culture (Reiter et al., 2020). Assessments of incarcerated individuals in solitary confinement are often conducted through a closed cell door, creating a more vulnerable environment that lacks privacy, and does not produce the most accurate assessments or encourage an incarcerated individuals to fully disclose their conditions (Grassian, 2006). This ought to influence how mental health professionals approach assessments, and how they consider a diagnosis and treatment path for patients in this group.

Aside from being prepared to respond to the impacts of solitary confinement from a treatment standpoint, mental health professionals in incarceration settings must also recognize the vulnerabilities and risks for long-term damage associated with solitary confinement. Since existing mental illnesses are worsened by solitary confinement and place an increased vulnerability for damage in this group, mental health professionals working in prisons can use this information to recommend effective treatment and advocate for one's release from isolation. Given that the risk for long-term damage from confinement increases after ten days, mental health professionals can also use this to stress the urgency to remove individuals from isolation to prevent such damage before this time frame passes (Cloud et al., 2015). This also specifies a crucial time frame for when an assessment should be conducted and when a mental health professional should be in contact with people in isolation. There is a responsibility on behalf of mental health professionals in incarceration settings to advocate for this mitigation of damages from solitary confinement, knowing the high potential for lasting damage. Being able to conduct accurate assessments in prison facilities further influences a mental health professional's ability to work to mitigate damages from solitary confinement. The practice of conducting more timely and reliable assessments is crucial to reduce harm and should be a priority of mental health professionals within incarceration facilities to allow for this proper treatment and mitigation of the impacts of confinement to occur as much as possible.

In addition to the barriers to treatment that exist in American society, many obstacles also exist in receiving treatment within incarceration settings. In many cases, incarcerated individuals are required to pay co-pays in prisons in order to receive treatment, which is not always possible for all people needing treatment (APA, 2014). Budget cuts within private prisons, which account for at least 10% of incarceration facilities, can also create gaps in treatment, as well as its quality (APA, 2014). Overcrowding, as well as dismissiveness or distrust toward the claims of incarcerated individuals, can also result in additional gaps in care (Smith, 2013). These barriers to treatment present the strong possibility that many incarcerated individuals did not receive quality, effective, or timely treatment, especially when combined with any hesitance on behalf of an incarcerated individual to disclose symptoms. This presents important contextual items to mental health professionals, in that they are encountering a vulnerable population with high rates of mental illness that typically lacked health insurance and access to effective health care outside of prison, and face further barriers to treatment in prison, where the inherent environment and common prison practices create these additional serious mental health risks (Smith, 2013). Aside from barriers to treatment that occur before and during incarceration, access to treatment post-release proves to continue to be difficult for people who have faced incarceration. It is common for incarcerated individuals with mental illness who do receive treatment in prison to deviate from medication routines after release (Smith, 2013). Mental health professionals ought to be aware of the inconsistent pattern of treatment that is likely to exist within this population, considering the factors that decrease their access to care before, during, and after incarceration.

Characteristics of the prison environment, prevalence of violence and sexual assault, as well as the use of solitary confinement, pose additional risks that worsen existing mental health conditions, as well as produce new symptoms within those who are incarcerated (Smith, 2013). While also leading the incarcerated prison population in the world, the United States also has the highest population of people in solitary confinement (Cloud et al., 2015). Reiter et al. (2020) had published research noting the prevalence and impacts of solitary confinement in the United States. Interviews and assessments were conducted with over 100 in solitary confinement (Reiter et al., 2020). In addition to psychometric measures, these assessments also included a review of medical and disciplinary records (Reiter et al., 2020). These findings highlight the common and detrimental effects of solitary confinement on a person's mental health and note the persistence of such symptoms that include severe anxiety, depression, hallucinations, paranoia, and severe sensory sensitivities (Reiter et al., 2020). This indicates the mental health risks and impacts associated with solitary confinement and is a notable study due to subsequent comparative follow-up interviews, which show the ongoing nature of these impacts, which makes these findings specifically compelling to show the related clinical implications (Reiter et al., 2020). Additional observations of those in solitary confinement in the 1990s at Pelican State Prison in California mirrored these findings and concluded that those with mental health conditions are more likely to be placed in solitary confinement (Grassian, 2006). These findings highlight the mental health risks of prison environments, as well as the dangers of using solitary confinement, especially with consideration to the treatment gaps and prevalence of mental illness in prison facilities.

Policy Implications

Establishing that the impacts of solitary confinement are common, severe, lasting, and far-reaching leads to questions about the ethical nature of using solitary confinement. Furthermore, this dilemma can be extended to general incarceration in the United States when considering the design and nature of prisons in America that are isolating and depriving, and thus produce conditions that can lead to lasting deterioration of an incarcerated individual's mental health. Arguments can be made that solitary confinement falls into the category of cruel and unusual punishment, while the design of prisons and use of isolation in America has roots in a previously forced monastic lifestyle that is contrary to the ideals of reform and rehabilitation (Davis, 2003). One cannot be rehabilitated and reformed to effectively function in society if their incarceration is permanently detrimental to their psychological health through solitary confinement and the isolating nature of prison facilities. The history, widespread use, and extraordinary impacts of solitary confinement imply a need for policy changes to reflect an acknowledgment of the damages associated with its use to either significantly limit or abolish its use altogether. There is a lack of policy to limit the duration of solitary confinement on the federal level and within 19 states, where incarcerated individuals can be held in isolation for indefinite time frames (Cloud et al., 2015). This is despite consistent research that has concluded that solitary confinement is likely to inflict permanent psychological damage after ten days (Cloud et al., 2015). In addition to the pressing need for policies to reflect limitations on solitary confinement within this range, there is a demand to re-examine the conditions under which an incarcerated individuals is placed in solitary confinement. Most incarcerated individuals placed in solitary confinement do not pose risks to the general prison population or staff and instead are isolated in such harsh and damaging conditions for punitive reasons such as talking back, smoking, or failing to return a meal tray (Cloud et al., 2015). The practice of the punitive use of isolation is reminiscent of the ways that mandatory minimums were established for small drug offenses, attributing to the substantial rise in incarceration since the 1980s (Shjarback & Young, 2017). The overlap in the extremity of the punishment for seemingly small offenses that can lead to lasting impacts in the form of incarceration, and psychologically through isolation reveal a problematic theme in the criminal justice system. Preventing such unnecessary, frivolous, isolation and incarceration would promote public health and prevent irreversible damage upon incarcerated individuals that would follow them throughout the rest of their lives post-release.

Given the barriers that exist to mental health treatment inside and outside of incarceration settings, there is a need for policies to expand access and coverage for mental health care, as well as alternatives to incarceration. Considering the prevalence of mental illness in prisons, barriers to treatment should be removed, such as required co-pays for visits that deter incarcerated individuals from receiving care (APA, 2014). Obstacles to treatment in the form of assessments and health care visits through a cell door or locked cage deprive incarcerated individuals of the dignity of privacy and comfort (Reiter et al., 2020). Policies on the facilitation of assessments and care ought to acknowledge the impacts this has on obtaining accurate assessments and preventing the disclosure of illness (Reiter et al., 2020). Exclusions to mental health treatment and the lack of adequate and available community care places the most vulnerable individuals at risk for interactions with law enforcement, and thus incarceration and isolation in the criminal justice system (Onah, 2018). Expanded access to treatment and alternatives to incarceration through mental health and drug courts could provide effective pathways to affirm the lives and well-being of those with mental health conditions and prevent further damage from being inflicted by incarceration and solitary confinement. Given the high representation of those with mental health conditions in prison and solitary confinement in America, such policies to expand health care and offer alternatives to incarceration could create pathways to challenging the very system of mass incarceration.

Policymakers could redesign prison systems to promote positive family relationships and child welfare. One area for improvement is visitation policies, as many families experience unfavorable conditions that are often hostile and intimidating, discouraging future contact (Arditti, 2012). For instance, visitation practices can disproportionately penalize minority groups due to unequal sentencing and biased behavioral evaluations (Cochran et al., 2017). This dynamic also significantly impacts child development, as the absence of an active father figure places additional emotional and financial strain on mothers, who must assume both parental roles (Bruns, 2019). In addressing the emotional and financial burdens on women with incarcerated partners, policymakers should ensure that immediate psychological and financial support is available. Additionally, families should be informed about how to access counseling services and emergency assistance, for example, parenting programs, including relationship counseling, have been shown to strengthen family bonds after incarceration (Lindquist et al., 2020). Similarly, prison programs that provide employment opportunities for incarcerated fathers could be expanded to offer child support during incarceration, reducing the economic burden on families. Policies could also prioritize consistent child support payments, ensuring that these payments take precedence over government debts (Geller et al., 2011). Additionally, programs that increase incentives, such as tax breaks, for hiring formerly incarcerated individuals could contribute to shared parental responsibilities.

Policy reforms could also be implemented at a broader, systemic level within corrections. Expanding social welfare in ways that intersect with correctional policies could benefit both incarcerated individuals and their communities (Lee et al., 2016). This might include sentencing reforms aimed at reducing the prison population while maintaining public safety (Wildeman & Western, 2010). For example, reforming post-incarceration supervision, such as parole and probation, could address the diverse social, economic, health, and psychological needs of individuals (Blankenship et al., 2018). It is well-documented that when individuals return to environments with limited resources, economic disadvantages, high crime rates, and restrictive correctional policies, they are more likely to re-enter the prison system (Lee et al., 2016). Minoritized communities, in particular, often experience heightened police surveillance, leading to skewed crime rates, community unrest, and increased stress-related health issues (Blankenship et al., 2018). Current correctional policies not only impact individuals but also have far-reaching effects on communities, making it a broader social issue. Therefore, addressing the specific needs of communities and understanding the intersection of the criminal justice system can help establish policies that are more equitable and promote both individual and societal well-being.

Future Research Directions

The clinical implications of the impacts that solitary confinement and incarceration have on the mental health of incarcerated individuals indicate a need for more research on effective psychological assessments that can be used to reveal damage incurred from solitary confinement, as well as properly assess the condition of those in prison. If the collection of symptoms that result from solitary confinement is not necessarily indicative of a specific existing mental illness, this complicates the process of assessing, diagnosing, and treating patients who are or have been incarcerated (Grassian, 2006). The Brief Psychiatric Rating Scale (BPRS) is often used to conduct research within incarceration settings, including solitary confinement units (Reiter et al., 2020). While it is effective at recognizing the presence of mental illness, it was initially designed to document changes in patients in psychiatric hospitals over time, as well as note the severity of one's symptoms (Reiter et al., 2020). In order to establish and increase reliability in assessing those in solitary confinement, the BPRS is combined with additional questionnaires, interviews, as well as the review of medical records upon consent (Reiter et al., 2020). This specifies a need for assessments that are designed specifically to detect the effects of solitary confinement from not only just a research perspective, but a practical treatment one. Research is needed in not only developing and testing such an assessment, but also in determining the effectiveness of other existing assessments that are commonly used.

Considering that assessments are not always held in private settings within confinement facilities and thus influence the nature of responses given by incarcerated individuals, research must also be done to evaluate the ways that the assessment approach and environment inform the validity of any assessment type conducted. Evaluating the effectiveness of an assessment, as well as developing assessments that are built to detect the impacts of solitary confinement, must include controlled environments where researchers and clinicians can work with incarcerated people in a setting that offers comfort and consideration for their safety and well-being. This must also translate to the application of such assessments for treatment purposes. Conducting assessments through locked doors, while incarcerated individuals are locked within small cages, or within settings that lack privacy, as they often are, will undermine any assessment method, as well as obscure the development of any new methods and research (Cloud et al., 2015). Reinforcing the most effective assessment approaches and methods in this population is necessary to accurately identify the scale of the damage from solitary confinement and also provide adequate treatment. Such approaches can also result in better assessments for all people in prison.

While much research has been conducted to reinforce the ways that solitary confinement is likely to have lasting impacts on an individual after ten days, which includes an assortment of psychological symptoms, additional research could also expand upon the ways that the use of solitary confinement further impacts the livelihood of formerly incarcerated individuals beyond the set of symptoms that they experience (Cloud et al., 2015). Incarceration affects the future employability of an individual and creates barriers for obtaining employment and accruing wealth post-release (Davis, 2003). Combining the existing obstacles to employment for people who were formerly incarcerated with common effects of solitary confinement that include persisting PTSD, social adjustment issues, sensory sensitivity, anxiety, and depression could substantially inhibit one's ability to function in a workplace and maintain employment (Cloud et al., 2015). Given the extent to which people are incarcerated in the United States and the extensive use of solitary confinement, in many cases without any limitations on the length of isolation, such impacts could be widespread (Cloud et al., 2015). Further research that leads to more detailed conclusions and findings about the ways that the use and impacts of solitary confinement could affect adjustment to society after prison, future employability, cycles of poverty, and risks for future reincarceration is necessary to fully understand the consequences of isolation in the prison system. Such findings could act as a further impetus and reason to reimagine the historic prison design in America that is isolating in nature, as well as significantly limit, reframe, or end the use of solitary confinement altogether.

Future research could also influence and direct considerations for alternatives to solitary confinement. Psychological impacts of solitary confinement mirror the effects of sensory deprivation (Grassian, 2006). Solitary confinement generally involves an extreme lack of proper stimulation, access to programming, or adequate human interactions (APA, 2014). If an incarcerated individual absolutely must be separated and isolated due to a legitimate safety concern, research is needed to explore ways to eliminate psychological damage from this isolation. Studying any possible potential to provide adequate stimulation, access to programming, and meaningful human interaction while in separation to prevent symptoms and damages associated with solitary confinement could reframe the use and standards of this widespread correctional practice.

References

American Psychological Association. (2014, October). *Incarceration nation*. Monitor on Psychology. Retrieved from https://www.apa.org/monitor/2014/10/incarceration

Arditti, J. (2012). *Parental incarceration and the family: Psychological and social effects of imprisonment on children, parents, and caregivers*. New York University Press. https://doi.org/10.18574/nyu/9780814705131.001.0001

Blankenship, K., Gonzalez, A., Keene, D., Groves, A., & Rosenberg, A. (2018, October). Mass incarceration, race inequality, and health: Expanding concepts and assessing impacts on well-being. *Social Science and Medicine, 215*, 45–52. https://doi.org/10.1016/j.socscimed.2018.08.042

Blomberg, T., Bales, W., Mann, K., Piquero, A., & Berk, R. (2011). Incarceration, education and transition from delinquency. *Elsevier*. https://doi.org/10.1016/j.jcrimjus.2011.04.003

Bruns, A. (2019). The third shift: Multiple job holding and the incarceration of women's partners. *Social Science Research, 80*. https://doi.org/10.1016/j.ssresearch.2018.12.024

Camp, S., & Gaes, G. (2001, September). *Growth and quality of U.S. private prisons: Evidence from a national survey*. Federal Bureau of Prisons. Retrieved from https://www.bop.gov/resources/research_projects/published_reports/pub_vs_priv/oreprres_note.pdf

Cloud, D. H., Drucker, E., Browne, A., & Parsons, J. (2015, January). Public health and solitary confinement in the United States. *American Journal of Public Health*. Retrieved from https://www.ncbi.nlm.nih.gov/pmc/articles/PMC4265928/

Cochran, J., Toman, E., Mears, D., & Bales, W. (2017, April). Solitary confinement as punishment: Examining in-prison sanctioning disparities. *Justice Quarterly, 35*(3). https://doi.org/10.1080/07418825.2017.1308541

Davis, A. (2003). *Are prisons obsolete?* Seven Stories Press.

Foucault, M. (1975). *Discipline & punish: The birth of the prison*. Knopf Doubleday Publishing Group.

Geller, A. (2013). Paternal Incarceration and Father-Child Contact in Fragile Families. *Journal of Marriage and Family, 75*(5), 1288–1303. https://doi.org/10.1111/jomf.12056

Goodman, N. (1934). *Benjamin rush: Physician and citizen 1746–1813*. University of Pennsylvania Press.

Grassian, S. (2006, January). Psychiatric effects of solitary confinement. *Washington University Journal of Law and Policy*. Retrieved from https://openscholarship.wustl.edu/cgi/viewcontent.cgi?article=1362&context=law_journal_law_policy

Human Rights Watch (2014). *World report 2014*. Retrieved from https://www.hrw.org/world-report/2014

Jefferson, T. (1779). 64. *A bill for proportioning crimes and punishments in cases heretofore capital*. Retrieved from https://founders.archives.gov/documents/Jefferson/01-02-02-0132-0004-0064

Lee, H., Wildeman, C., Wang, E. A., Matusko, N., & Jackson, J. S. (2016). A heavy burden: The cardiovascular health consequences of having a family member incarcerated. *American Journal of Public Health, 104*(3), 421–427. https://doi.org/10.2105/AJPH.2013.301504

Lindquist, C. H., McKay, T. E., & Bir, A. (2020). Lessons from the Multi-Site Family Study of Incarceration, Parenting, and Partnering. In P. K. Lattimore, B. M. Huebner, & F. S. Taxman (Eds.), *Handbook on Moving Corrections and Sentencing Forward: Building on the Record* (pp. 187–215). Routledge.

Lindsey, A., Mears, D., & Cochran, J. (2016). The privatization debate: A conceptual framework for improving (public and private) corrections. *Journal of Contemporary Criminal Justice, 32*(4). https://doi.org/10.1177/1043986216660006

Mate, G. (1999). *Scattered minds: The origins and healing of attention deficit disorder*. Avery Publishing.

McLennan, R. (2009). *The crisis of imprisonment. Protest, politics and the making of the American penal state (1776–1941)*. Cambridge University Press. https://doi.org/10.4000/chs.1156

Morgan, E., Rivara, F., Ta, M., Grossman, D., Jones, K., & Rowhani-Rahbar, A. (2022, January). Incarceration and subsequent risk of suicide: A statewide cohort study. *National Library of Medicine, 52*(3). https://doi.org/10.1111/sltb.12834

Onah, M. E. (2018). The patient-to-prisoner pipeline: The Imd Exclusion's adverse impact on mass incarceration in United States. *American Journal of Law & Medicine, 44*(1), 119–144. https://doi.org/10.1177/0098858818763818

Reiter, K., Ventura, J., Lovell, D., Augustine, D., Barragan, M., Blair, T., Chesnut, K., Dashtgard, P., Gonzalez, G., Pifer, N., & Strong, J. (2020). Psychological distress in solitary confinement: Symptoms, severity, and prevalence in the United States, 2017–2018. *American Journal of Public Health, 110*(S1). https://doi.org/10.2105/ajph.2019.305375

Shjarback, J. A., & Young, J. T. (2017). The "tough on crime" competition: A network approach to understanding the social mechanisms leading to federal crime control legislation in the United States from 1973–2014. *American Journal of Criminal Justice, 43*(2), 197–221. https://doi.org/10.1007/s12103-017-9395-5

Smith, A. (2013). *Health and incarceration: A workshop summary*. National Academy Press.

Swanson, C., Lee, C., Sansone, F., & Tatum, K. (2013, August). Incarcerated fathers and their children: Perceptions of barriers to their relationships. *Sage Journals: The Prison Journal, 93*(4). https://doi.org/10.1177/0032885513501024

Tadros, E., Presley, S., & Guzman, Y. (2023). "Who Are You Really Punishing?": Mothers' experiences with an incarcerated son. *Crime & Delinquency, 0*(0). https://doi.org/10.1177/00111287221146544

Tadros, E., Schleiden, C., Jenkins, L., & Aguirre, N. (2021). The experiences of marriage and family therapists working in incarcerated settings. *American Journal of Family Therapy, 49*(5), 461–479. https://doi.org/10.1080/01926187.2020.1834469

Wildeman, C., & Western, B. (2010). Incarceration in fragile families. *The Future of Children, 20*(2), 157–177. https://www.jstor.org/stable/20773699

Chapter 8

Ethical Considerations

Yenitza Z. Guzman, Annemarie Sohn and Eman Tadros

Historically, incarcerated individuals have been a vulnerable population, often exploited by researchers and physicians due to their accessibility (Dalen & Jones, 2010). Ethical and legal issues are especially important for clinicians in correctional settings, including those in Marriage and Family Therapy (MFT). MFT employs contemporary therapeutic strategies and theories to assist couples and families in addressing and overcoming maladaptive behaviors (American Association for Marriage and Family Therapy [AAMFT], 2015). Incarcerated settings pose unique challenges, making it essential for therapists to understand their ethical and legal responsibilities while upholding the rights of incarcerated individuals and their families.

MFTs should be vigilant in their pursuit of knowledge regarding ethical and legal issues, as even well-intended actions can cause harm. They must abide by ethical codes and legal statutes, and practice according to the highest standards possible. This chapter explores ethical and logistical considerations when working with the incarcerated population, including informed consent, confidentiality, and research considerations.

Ethical Considerations: ACA Counseling Ethics

To guard against making unethical decisions, MFTs use multiple resources. The most prevalent aid is the American Counseling Association's (ACA) Code of Ethics. According to ACA (2014) Code of Ethics, there are six ethical principles that are the foundation for ethical behavior and decision-making: autonomy, nonmaleficence, beneficence, justice, fidelity, and veracity.

1 *Autonomy* – concerning a person's right to make his or her own choices and to be treated with respect, including respect for one's cultural and individual differences.
2 *Nonmaleficence* – capturing in the Hippocratic oath of "Above all, do no harm."

DOI: 10.4324/9781003542940-8

3 *Beneficence* – concerning the well-being of others and optimizing benefits over risks.
4 *Justice* – concerning fairness in distributing risks, benefits, and costs.
5 *Fidelity* – concerning keeping promises and taking responsibility for one's work with others.
6 *Veracity* – concerning being truthful with individuals with whom one comes in contact.

The ACA Code of Ethics (2024) gives an overview for counselors across populations. However, therapists working with this protected population must especially apply these principles from the perspective of their clients' and families' specific needs. Additional guidelines from CACREP (2016), ACES (2016), and NBCC (2016) emphasize multicultural competencies. Mental health practitioners must consider social, cultural, and political realities that impact marginalized clients. These factors directly affect their sense of belonging, which is a core principle in psychology (Tummala-Narra, 2015). While the ACA Code of Ethics offers broad guidance, therapists working with protected populations should be familiar with the AAMFT Code of Ethics. The following section highlights key ethical considerations.

AAMFT Ethical Considerations

To ensure client well-being and professional conduct, MFTs must follow the AAMFT Code of Ethics, which may set higher standards than state laws and regulations (AAMFT, 2015). Working with incarcerated individuals and their families presents unique challenges that require a nuanced understanding of systemic therapy and ethics.

There are presently 128 competences for MFTs, categorized into six basic domains and five secondary areas. The fundamental core competences include admission to treatment, clinical assessment and diagnosis, treatment planning and case management, therapeutic treatments, legal considerations, ethics, and standards, as well as research and program evaluation (AAMFT, 2004). The secondary core abilities include conceptual, perceptual, executive, evaluative, and professional (AAMFT, 2004). A code of ethics exists for MFTs reflecting the fundamental ideals of the AAMFT and comprising nine criteria they adhere to. The nine standards of the code of ethics include: responsibility to clients, confidentiality, professional competence and integrity, responsibility to students and supervisees, research and publication, technology-assisted professional services, professional evaluations, financial arrangements, and advertising (AAMFT, 2015). The fundamental and secondary core competencies, together with ethical standards, are established to guarantee the quality of work and the ethical conduct that MFTs must adhere to effectively.

The non-discrimination principle, Standard 1.1, is critical for MFTs to follow (AAMFT, 2015), even if the AAMFT does not particularly outline rules for working with minoritized communities. According to Finney et al. (2020), therapists should not discriminate based on a client's race, ethnicity, or socioeconomic background. The AAMFT recently strengthened its commitment to inclusivity with a Gender-Affirming Care Position Statement approved by the Board of Directors in October 2024, which emphasizes the need for affirming, culturally attuned care for trans, nonbinary, and gender-expansive individuals and their families, including children and youth (AAMFT, 2024). For MFTs to be effective, they must recognize and confront the political, cultural, and social factors that challenge individuals with marginalized identities' sense of belonging (Tummala-Narra, 2015). MFTs must recognize the unique dynamics in families affected by incarceration and make every effort to understand and address these complexities in order to facilitate clinical work with incarcerated individuals, especially because there are no defined procedures to do so.

Adherence to provincial or state laws, confidentiality, technological training, and correct documentation are all outlined in the AAMFT Code of Ethics (AAMFT, 2015). Standard 1.2 elucidates the concept of informed consent and emphasizes the significance of client understanding (AAMFT, 2015). However, research on the ethical and legal guidelines for technology use in MFT found that state laws and regulations are limited, with minimal mention of technology. In fact, seven states had no mention of technology at all (Pennington et al., 2017). Given the potential literacy difficulties faced by jailed individuals, it is crucial to establish a continuous process of informed consent for them and their family to ensure full understanding (Barnett & Kolmes, 2016). Obstacles like this can serve as hindrances that can be reduced with the assistance of therapists who remain knowledgeable about such issues.

Obtaining high-quality services while in prison is crucial for addressing both pre-existing and newly arising problems, as well as minimizing the health hazards individuals encounter upon reintegrating into society (Canada et al., 2022). Further, it is vital to uphold client autonomy in decision-making, as outlined in Standard 1.8. This is particularly critical when addressing matters such as visitation, communication with family members, and the process of reintegrating into society after release (AAMFT, 2015). Therapists should assist incarcerated clients in making well-informed choices regarding their relationships and future decisions.

The significance of confidentiality concerns, Standard 2, is particularly emphasized in working in incarcerated settings. MFTs are required to effectively convey information regarding the level of confidentiality, the conditions under which disclosure may occur, and the legal limitations involved (AAMFT, 2015). To guarantee client access to documents, therapists must carefully evaluate the advantages and disadvantages while also documenting any limitations in treatment.

In accordance with Standard 3.3 of the AAMFT Code of Ethics, MFTs are expected to seek support or consultation as necessary (AAMFT, 2015). Therefore, MFTs who work with incarcerated individuals are required to seek supervision or advice to effectively treat their clients. According to the code, MFTs are required to uphold confidentiality and professional obligations, as stated in Standard 6.3 (AAMFT, 2015; Caldwell, 2016). Therefore, safeguarding client's identifiable information is paramount in protecting incarcerated individuals who also possess intersecting identities that are associated with other vulnerable populations.

More MFTs should practice integrity and clear communication as a priority to maintain their professional integrity, especially in light of recent research showing that incarcerated populations benefit greatly from couple and family therapy (Tadros et al., 2019, 2020). Professional counselors need to continue efforts to develop, maintain and adjust a professional identity. With a focus on overall wellness, counselors look to establish and maintain a cohesive, unified, professional identity that addresses the needs of clients developmentally, mentally, emotionally, and in their day-to-day lives (Oramas, 2017). Concerning potential conflicts of interest, the AAMFT addresses them in Standard 3.4 (2015). Therapists are expected to skillfully balance their clients' needs with the constraints of their institution to meet these criteria (AAMFT, 2015). This can be achieved by MFTs acquiring and actively seeking knowledge about the distinct difficulties encountered by individuals in the criminal justice system and obtaining suitable training to assure their proficiency in handling these matters.

Commitment to Cultural Responsiveness

While the AAMFT website includes a diversity statement, it falls short of providing substantive guidance for integrating multicultural frameworks into therapeutic practice, highlighting the necessity for a more comprehensive approach to understanding and evaluating the complex interpersonal dynamics between therapists and clients. Multicultural "competencies" aren't an additional subspecialty; rather, they should be integrated into therapy regardless of population, facility, clinician, or theoretical orientation. Culturally informed care could assist in promoting services to diverse clients, which would be especially accommodating to incarcerated individuals and their families (Tadros et al., 2019). Yet, multicultural orientation (MCO) is proposed as a more extensive framework for comprehending and evaluating the multicultural foundations of the intricate interpersonal dynamics between therapists and clients (Tadros & Owens, 2021). Interestingly, ethical issues in relation to multicultural counseling are most frequent in the lack of competence from mental health professionals (Pack-Brown et al., 2008). Therefore, this is a necessity when working with a particularly racially and ethnically diverse population, such as those who are incarcerated.

General Considerations

Protected Population

A "vulnerable population" is a disadvantaged community subgroup that is unable to make informed decisions, protect themselves from inherent or intended hazards, or protect their own interests (Aday, 2002). Studying protected populations, including incarcerated individuals, gives rise to notable ethical considerations because of their increased susceptibility. Individuals who are incarcerated are classified as a protected group due to their restricted independence, vulnerability to manipulation, and historical background of being used in studies. Historical instances of unethical research within prisons have led to stringent oversight and heightened ethical scrutiny to safeguard participants' rights and well-being.

Incarcerated individuals navigate environments defined by strict control and limited autonomy, where decision-making power rests largely with authority figures. Within this context, powerlessness becomes a central concern, reflecting a lack of agency that can impact how individuals perceive and respond to situations involving consent. The powerlessness experienced by incarcerated individuals mirrors the loss of control often associated with trauma. This connection is significant given the higher prevalence of trauma and PTSD among incarcerated populations compared to the general public (Haney, 2012). The dynamic of powerlessness becomes key to observe in research settings, as a limited understanding of personal rights and fear of retaliation can create coercive conditions.

Challenges of Working with a Protected Population

Due to the prevalence of unethical research undertaken in prison settings throughout history, researchers frequently have apprehension when considering conducting studies with this population. Moser et al. (2004) compared 30 incarcerated individuals with mental health illnesses to 30 healthy controls in terms of their capacity to give informed consent for a hypothetical medication trial, susceptibility to coercion, neuropsychological functioning, and other psychiatric symptoms.

Results revealed that the vast majority of individuals had sufficient consent capacity, while others obtained lower scores on quantitative assessments of decisional capacity (Moser et al, 2004). Participants mentioned several motivations, including the need to alleviate boredom, socialize with new individuals, demonstrate cooperation, and contribute to society, as motives for participation. The study determined that while a significant number of incarcerated individuals, struggling with mental health, are capable of providing informed consensus for research, the lower scores in decisional competence underscore the importance of exercising additional caution during the consent procedure. The impact of the environment on individuals' choices to participate implies an absence of force but necessitates careful ethical deliberation to prevent excessive protection of this group.

Balancing Ethical Safeguards and Research Opportunities for Incarcerated Populations

Excessive protection of incarcerated populations can present substantial difficulties. Concerns about the ethical engagement of incarcerated individuals in research encompass perceived coercion by authorities, economic constraints, and the inherent hazards associated with participating in trials. Studies argue for enhanced oversight and the inclusion of the lived experiences of incarcerated individuals to mitigate these issues (Coughlin et al., 2016). The ethical obligation is to strike a balance between safeguarding and the necessity for research that has the potential to be advantageous for this marginalized population (Emanuel et al., 2000). Although the purpose is to protect their rights and well-being, severe limitations may unintentionally impede their independence and chances to engage in possibly advantageous research. This excessive shielding can result in an absence of inclusion in research, consequently preventing these folks from progressions that could enhance their health and overall welfare (Ako et al., 2020). Finding a balance between safety and autonomy is the key to upholding ethical norms without placing unwarranted restrictions on the ability of incarcerated individuals to participate in research.

There are many who contend that the strict safeguards might result in excessive protection for this group, potentially impeding significant research that could be advantageous for incarcerated persons and society as a whole. To ensure that incarcerated individuals are not unfairly excluded from research opportunities or exploited, ethical research practices must strike a balance between participant protection and the advancement of scientific knowledge (Ako et al., 2020).

Researchers can engage those incarcerated in research ethically by applying exacting ethical standards and promoting transparent communication. Although ethical concerns about coercion often limit direct compensation for participation in incarcerated settings (Eldridge et al., 2011), it is important for future research to also explore ways to empower research participants by involving them actively in the development, data collection, and analysis of research. This approach allows for breakthroughs in health and social sciences while upholding participants' rights and ensuring their protection.

Informed Consent and Research

While mental health research conducted within the context of incarceration has contributed valuable insights, it is crucial to acknowledge its potential harm to incarcerated individuals. Incarcerated individuals have been exploited in the past by researchers in order to serve the general population (Gostin et al., 2007). Obtaining informed consent, especially when conducting research, should be a primary responsibility of any therapist, especially those working with incarcerated populations.

Informed Consent in Research with Incarcerated Populations

Obtaining informed consent and voluntary participation are essential components of ethical research conduct, particularly when conducting studies involving vulnerable groups like incarcerated individuals. Incarcerated individuals face a myriad of challenges that may impact their ability to provide truly informed consent including low educational attainment, limited literacy, high rates of mental illness, cognitive impairments, and sensory deficits (Ahalt et al., 2018). Moreover, the aging prison population introduces additional complexities, as age-related conditions such as dementia may further impede comprehension (Ahalt et al., 2018).

In the context of research involving incarcerated populations, informed consent refers to the systematic provision of thorough and understandable information to participants regarding the study's goal, procedures, potential dangers and benefits, as well as their rights as participants. This procedure guarantees that individuals have the ability to make a deliberate and well-informed choice on their participation. In research involving incarcerated populations, informed consent must ensure that the potential benefits of participation outweigh the risks (Institute of Medicine [US] Committee on Ethical Considerations for Revisions to DHHS Regulations for Protection of Prisoners Involved in Research, 2007). Even seemingly harmless interview questions can provoke emotional or psychological distress, and such risks should only be allowed if they are balanced by a corresponding benefit to the incarcerated individuals involved (Institute of Medicine [US] Committee on Ethical Considerations for Revisions to DHHS Regulations for Protection of Prisoners Involved in Research, 2007). This thorough risk assessment is essential to ensuring ethical integrity in the research process.

Guidelines stipulate that research involving incarcerated individuals must undergo extra scrutiny, and IRBs must include representation from the incarcerated population (Crane et al., 2013). Crane et al. (2013) emphasize the significance of making sure that participants grasp the nature of their involvement and willingly consent to participate in research initiatives. In gaining valid informed consent from incarcerated individuals, it can be particularly challenging because of their vulnerable status and the potential effect of external circumstances, such as legal mandates, parole or correctional programming decisions (National Institute of Justice, 2012).

Ethical Progression and Guidelines

The development of ethical standards in research has been influenced by a historical context of unethical research methods. The Nuremberg Code and subsequent declarations, such as the Declaration of Helsinki, highlighted the significance of voluntary involvement and informed consent (Crane et al., 2013). To ensure the ethical conduct of research involving human participants, Institutional Review Boards (IRBs) were established. The concept of informed consent has gradually developed to include aspects such as understanding, willingness, and the communication of potential risks and benefits.

The American Psychological Association (APA) has been instrumental in establishing ethical guidelines for psychologists engaged in human research. According to the APA's Ethical Principles of Psychologists and Code of Conduct, researchers are required to give participants thorough information, which includes explaining the objective of the research, discussing potential risks and benefits, and informing participants of their right to withdraw from the study (Crane et al., 2013). Furthermore, the APA highlights the need for upholding the autonomy and rights of individuals involved in research.

The ethical imperative to ensure informed consent among incarcerated individuals is underscored by the inherent power differentials and constraints within correctional settings. Ahalt et al. (2018) emphasize the importance of upholding ethical standards in research with incarcerated populations, highlighting the necessity for additional safeguards to protect participants' autonomy and ensure discernment of research risks and benefits. Yet, there is a significant level of comprehension around communication, privacy, and therapy, which is prevalent among many individuals. Ensuring the rights, safety, data privacy, and confidentiality of these vulnerable individuals is a significant component of ethical research methods. Legal frameworks and regulations are in place to guarantee these protections and are regularly monitored by appropriate authorities.

Recommendations for Enhancing Informed Consent

Traditional approaches to obtaining informed consent, such as lengthy consent forms written at a high reading level, may not adequately address the urgent needs of incarcerated individuals. Ahalt et al. (2018) suggest that while efforts have been made to protect against coercion and undue influence, strategies to ensure awareness of informed consent are relatively limited. Informed consent processes for incarcerated populations often lack accessibility due to systemic and situational barriers (Esposito et al., 2024). Therefore, enhancing informed consent for incarcerated populations requires a thoughtful, ethical approach that prioritizes autonomy, clarity, and respect for participants' and clients' rights.

Consent forms frequently use complex or ambiguous language, including legal and technical jargon that can be difficult for individuals with lower literacy levels to understand (Simonds et al., 2017). Additionally, forms may fail to account for cultural or linguistic diversity, further complicating comprehension (Goodman et al., 2013). A lack of transparency about rights can also pose significant challenges; incarcerated individuals may not fully understand their right to refuse participation or withdraw without consequences, and explanations of confidentiality often neglect to address the inherent limitations within correctional settings (Van Westendorp & Lierman, 2020). One approach could be to employ straightforward, unambiguous language in consent forms and research descriptions, avoiding jargon to guarantee that incarcerated individuals comprehensively grasp the research's nature, their rights, and the associated risks and benefits (Simonds et al., 2017).

Facilitating access to independent advocacy or legal representatives can enhance their autonomy and shield against pressure (Liu & Dipietro, 2016). Given the inherent power imbalance in correctional settings, it's important to be aware of how coercive forces – whether real or perceived – might impact the decision to participate in research. Overgeneralized approaches to consent often disregard the diverse cultural, educational, and personal backgrounds of incarcerated populations, failing to address their unique needs and concerns (Crutchfield & Weeks, 2015). To guarantee that the particular needs and experiences of those who are incarcerated are acknowledged and taken into consideration, cultural sensitivity is also necessary during the consent process (Jones et al., 2013). This multi-faceted approach to ensure continuous ethical oversight of the consent process makes it even more important to create an environment where individuals feel the ethical standards and empowerment of incarcerated people within research and practice.

Furthermore, informed consent is often treated as a one-time event rather than an ongoing process, leaving participants without opportunities to revisit or reassess their involvement (Tinkler et al., 2018). To address these barriers, systemic changes are needed, including simplifying consent language, providing consistent education on participants' rights, offering independent advocacy, and fostering culturally responsive communication. In adhering to rigorous consent procedures and implementing tailored strategies, researchers can uphold ethical standards and protect the rights and well-being of vulnerable participants in criminal justice settings (Crane et al., 2013). Further research is warranted to refine and optimize the informed consent process in this context.

Confidentiality

Confidentiality is another fundamental principle of ethical conduct in mental health services. One of the principles of caring for people, including those involved in the criminal justice system, adheres to ethics guidelines aimed at protecting the rights and dignity of incarcerated individuals (Eichelberger et al., 2023).

Ethical Considerations with Confidentiality

An essential challenge for healthcare personnel responsible for the well-being of incarcerated patients is acquiring and preserving their trust (Eichelberger et al., 2023). This population often harbors a deep-seated distrust toward the criminal justice system and may believe that healthcare workers are obligated to report to prison authorities, leading to perceptions of divided loyalties (Tadros et al., 2023a). The concept of double loyalty refers to healthcare staff's dual responsibility: caring for the patient's health and well-being while also being accountable to jail and legal authorities (Pont et al., 2012). This dual role can generate ethical, political, and interprofessional tensions, potentially harming patient-provider relationships and trust.

MFTs in correctional settings often face conflicts of dual loyalty, balancing their ethical obligations to clients with the demands of the correctional system. This dual role can complicate the maintenance of confidentiality. Practitioners must navigate these challenges by adhering to established ethical guidelines, such as those outlined by the American Association for Marriage and Family Therapy (AAMFT, 2015). According to the AAMFT Code of Ethics, maintaining client confidentiality is crucial; however, there are circumstances where breaches may be necessary, such as in cases of clear and imminent danger to the client or others.

Legal Requirements

Legal requirements significantly influence the boundaries of confidentiality in correctional settings. Different states have varying laws regarding confidentiality, and mental health practitioners must be well-versed in these regulations to fulfill their responsibilities effectively. Research indicates that legal guidelines for technology use in mental health treatment are often inadequate or nonexistent, with many states lacking specific regulations (Pennington et al., 2017). This legal ambiguity can extend to confidentiality issues, necessitating that practitioners rely on professional ethical standards and institutional policies to guide them.

Practical Challenges

Maintaining confidentiality within correctional environments presents several practical challenges. The physical setup of correctional facilities often does not support private communication between practitioners and clients, which can compromise confidentiality. Additionally, the presence of correctional officers (even if right outside the door) during sessions or the requirement to share certain information with correctional staff can further complicate efforts to uphold confidentiality (White et al., 2014). MFTs may also have issues with scheduling and time constraints when working with their clients in correctional facilities. Many therapy sessions can be limited, interrupted, or delayed due to overcrowding or security protocols, which may make it difficult to build a consistent therapeutic relationship. Also, there may be inadequate resources and bureaucratic limitations that may create additional barriers for ongoing mental health services (Canada et al., 2022).

Practical Applications

In practice, maintaining confidentiality involves several key actions. Clinicians should recognize that attending therapy is often a significant barrier for incarcerated clients and even more so for clients of racially and ethnically minoritized backgrounds, thus, they should address confidentiality concerns from the first session (Tadros et al., 2023b). Practitioners must clearly communicate the boundaries of confidentiality during the informed consent process, ensure that all discussions and records are kept private and secure, and be transparent about circumstances under which confidentiality might need to be breached, such as imminent harm to the client or others (AAMFT, 2015).

Continual training and ethical evaluation have become essential in guaranteeing that professionals maintain the utmost level of confidentiality and effectively handle any ethical dilemmas that may arise during their work (Pope, 2007). Consistent professional growth and strict compliance with updated ethical standards assist professionals in managing the intricacies of confidentiality in many contexts, such as correctional facilities. To effectively maintain the integrity of their practice and safeguard their clients' rights, practitioners must stay updated on current legal and ethical standards. This enables them to effectively navigate the complex relationship between client confidentiality and other professional obligations.

Strategies for Maintaining Confidentiality

To effectively manage confidentiality, mental health practitioners should employ several strategies. First, they should clearly communicate the limits of confidentiality to incarcerated clients during the informed consent process, discussing situations where confidentiality might be breached, such as threats to safety or legal requirements (AAMFT, 2015). Ensuring that clients understand these boundaries can enhance their willingness to share sensitive information, which is essential for effective therapy (AAMFT, 2015).

Second, respecting a client's confidentiality demonstrates a commitment to their autonomy and dignity, fostering a sense of security and mutual trust that is foundational to a therapeutic relationship (Peternelj-Taylor, 2004). The Committee on Ethical Considerations for Revisions to DHHS Regulations for Protection of Prisoners Involved in Research emphasizes that maintaining confidentiality has significance for preserving trust and respect for incarcerated individuals who may already experience vulnerability and exploitation (Pope, 2007). This trust, in turn, supports clients in feeling valued and respected, which is critical for their overall well-being and engagement in the treatment process (Peternelj-Taylor, 2004).

Third, practitioners should maintain detailed and secure records of all communications and decisions related to confidentiality, which protects both the client and the practitioner in case of future disputes (Pont et al., 2012) Comprehensive documentation serves multiple purposes. It not only ensures transparency but also provides a safeguard for both clients and practitioners in the event of future disputes or legal scrutiny. Accurate records help clarify the context and rationale for any decisions made concerning confidentiality, thereby protecting practitioners from potential legal or ethical challenges. Ensuring confidentiality helps alleviate fears among incarcerated individuals that sharing personal information could lead to negative consequences within the correctional system (White et al., 2014). Lastly, staff members should receive adequate training in the ethical and legal aspects of confidentiality and regular supervision to manage complex cases effectively (Aday & Farney, 2014).

Case Studies: Ethical Considerations in Therapy with an Incarcerated Individual

Case studies can be great tools to use when applying learning for MFTs. In what follows, you will find case studies for therapists working with an incarcerated individual.

Case Study Example #1

Alex Smith is a 40-year-old cis-gender white male serving a 15-year sentence for drug trafficking, currently serving the 8th year of his sentence. Alex grew up in a middle-class family but became estranged from them after getting involved in illegal activities. He has a history of substance abuse. Alex has been diagnosed with a major depressive disorder and has a history of suicidal ideation. He has been receiving medication and therapy in prison.

Alex requested therapy to deal with persistent depression, feelings of guilt and shame related to his criminal activities, and concerns about reentering society. He also expressed a desire to reconnect with his family, particularly his teenage daughter, whom he has not seen since his incarceration. He would like his therapist to support him with how and when to reach out to this family, including what exactly he needs to say to them to "get on their good side." What are some ethical considerations the therapist should be aware of?

This case underscores the importance of ethical vigilance in a correctional setting, where multiple interests and pressures may impact the therapeutic process. The therapist must understand the limits placed on Alex in terms of communicating with loved ones outside of the prison setting and encourage Alex to use what is in his control – his own words and feelings – to fully express himself. Alex's therapist must consistently prioritize his welfare, autonomy, and the ethical and legal guidelines of confidentiality and informed consent, as well as a clear adherence to professional standards of the counseling profession.

Case Study Example #2

Andrea is a 30-year old woman incarcerated for a two year sentence for a theft-related offense. She has a history of bipolar disorder and was prescribed medication before her incarceration, though she has struggled with adherence. Andrea expresses that she is interested in resuming her medication but feels uninformed and pressured to make medical decisions that she does not agree with. She becomes extremely erratic and paranoid as she describes that the facility's psychiatrist told her she must accept new medication or face disciplinary consequences that could include solitary confinement or loss of privileges.

The therapist in this case faces an ethical dilemma. The therapist wants to support Andrea and empathize with her situation so that she can feel empowered and respected. The therapist wants Andrea to feel informed and that she has autonomy over her medical decisions. However, Andrea seems to change her story and become very paranoid about how "everyone is out to get her." The therapist must navigate the tension between advocating for Andrea while avoiding interference with the facility's medical policies. What is the best course of action for this therapist?

This case illustrates the ethical challenges of informed consent and autonomy in a correctional setting, where incarcerated individuals face limited options. The therapist can focus on autonomy by ensuring that the client feels comfortable advocating for themselves and addressing their medical needs, while ensuring that they are in a healthy state of mind to do so. This case highlights the importance of helping incarcerated clients navigate complex healthcare decisions by fostering informed decision-making and self-advocacy skills.

Conclusion

Mental health professionals must consider a variety of ethical and logistical considerations when working with the incarcerated population. By upholding principles such as confidentiality, informed consent, and ethical guidelines, counselors can provide valuable support to incarcerated individuals as they work toward rehabilitation and reintegration into society. The therapeutic alliance is significantly strengthened when clients trust that their therapists will protect their confidentiality. This trust is critical for the success of therapeutic interventions, as research indicates that a strong therapeutic alliance correlates with better treatment outcomes (Norcross & Lambert, 2018). Adherence to legal and ethical standards regarding confidentiality reassures clients that their rights are respected, which is particularly important in correctional settings where clients may feel vulnerable and distrustful of authority figures (Pont et al., 2012). Confidentiality in these settings is a complex issue that requires practitioners to balance ethical principles, legal requirements, and practical challenges. By adhering to professional ethical guidelines, staying informed about relevant laws, and employing effective strategies, practitioners can navigate these challenges and provide ethically sound care to incarcerated individuals.

References

AAMFT. (2004). Core competencies for marriage and family therapists. https://www.aamft.org/Documents/COAMFTE/Accreditation%20Resources/MFT%20Co%20Competencies%20(December%202004).pdf

AAMFT. (2015). Code of ethics. American association for marriage and family therapy. https://www.aamft.org/Legal_Ethics/Code_of_Ethics.aspx.

Aday, L. A. (2002). *At risk in America: The health and health care needs of vulnerable populations in the United States* (Vol. 13). John Wiley & Sons.

Aday, R., & Farney, L. (2014). Malign neglect: assessing older women's health care experiences in prison. *Journal of Bioethical Inquiry*, *11*(3), 359–372. https://doi.org/10.1007/s11673-014-9561-0

Ahalt, C., Sudore, R., Bolano, M., Metzger, L., Darby, A. M., Williams, B. A., & Smith, A. K. (2018). "Teach-to-Goal" to better assess informed consent comprehension among incarcerated clinical research participants. *Ethics & Human Research*, *40*(6), 29–36.

Ako, T., Plugge, E., Mhlanga-Gunda, R., & Van Hout, M. C. (2020). Ethical guidance for health research in prisons in low- and middle-income countries: A scoping review. *Public Health*, *186*, 217–227. https://doi.org/10.1016/j.puhe.2020.07.008

American Association for Marriage and Family Therapy. (2015). AAMFT code of ethics. https://www.aamft.org/Legal_Ethics/Code_of_Ethics.aspx

American Association for Marriage and Family Therapy. (2024, October). Gender-affirming care position statement. https://www.aamft.org/AAMFT/About_AAMFT/Pos_on_couples.aspx

Barnett, J. E., & Kolmes, K. (2016). The practice of tele-mental health: Ethical, legal, and clinical issues for practitioners. *Practice Innovations, 1*(1), 53–66. https://doi.org/10.1037/pri0000014.

Caldwell, B. E. (2016). Ethics and supervision. In K. Jordan (Ed.), *Couple, marriage, and family therapy supervision* (pp. 151–168). Springer Publishing Company.

Canada, K., Barrenger, S., Bohrman, C., Banks, A., & Peketi, P. (2022). Multi-level barriers to prison mental health and physical health care for individuals with mental illnesses. *Frontiers in Psychiatry, 13*, 777124. https://doi.org/10.3389/fpsyt.2022.777124

Coughlin, S. S., Lewis, S. R., & Smith, S. A. (2016). Ethical and social issues in health research involving incarcerated people. *Journal of Health Care for the Poor and Underserved, 27*(2A), 18–28. https://doi.org/10.1353/hpu.2016.0053

Crane, C. A., Hawes, S. W., Mandel, D., & Easton, C. J. (2013). Informed consent: An ethical issue in conducting research with male partner violent offenders. *Ethics & Behavior, 23*(6), 477–488. https://doi.org/10.1080/10508422.2013.804795

Crutchfield, R. D., & Weeks, G. A. (2015). The effects of mass incarceration on communities of color. *Issues in Science and Technology, 32*(1), 45–61.

Dalen, K., & Jones, L. Ø. (2010). Ethical Monitoring: Conducting Research in a Prison Setting. *Research Ethics*, 6(1), 10–16. https://doi.org/10.1177/174701611000600103 (Original work published 2010).

Eichelberger, M., Wertli, M. M., & Tran, N. T. (2023). Equivalence of care, confidentiality, and professional independence must underpin the hospital care of individuals experiencing incarceration. *BMC Medical Ethics, 24*(1), 13. https://doi.org/10.1186/s12910-023-00891-3

Eldridge, G. D., Johnson, M. E., Brems, C., & Corey, S. L. (2011). Ethical challenges in conducting psychiatric or mental health research in correctional settings. *AJOB Primary Research, 2*(4), 42–51. https://doi.org/10.1080/21507716.2011.631964

Emanuel, E. J., Wendler, D., & Grady, C. (2000). What makes clinical research ethical? *JAMA*, 283(20), 2701–2711. https://doi.org/10.1001/jama.283.20.2701

Esposito, M., Szocik, K., Capasso, E., Chisari, M., Sessa, F., & Salerno, M. (2024). Respect for bioethical principles and human rights in prisons: A systematic review on the state of the art. *BMC Medical Ethics, 25*(1), 62. https://doi.org/10.1186/s12910-024-01049-5

Finney, N., Tadros, E., Pfeiffer, S., & Owens, D. (2020). Clinical implications for multi-racial individuals. *American Journal of Family Therapy, 48*(3), 271–282. https://doi.org/10.1080/01926187.2019.1709581

Goodman, M., Finnegan, R., Mohadjer, L., Krenzke, T., & Hogan, J. (2013). Literacy, Numeracy, and problem solving in technology-rich environments among US adults: Results from the program for the international assessment of adult competencies 2012. First Look. NCES 2014–008. National center for education statistics.

Gostin, L. O., Vanchieri, C. F., & Pope, A. M. (Eds.). (2007). *Ethical considerations for research involving prisoners.* National Academies Press. https://doi.org/10.17226/11692

Haney, C. (2012). Prison effects in the era of mass incarceration. *The Prison Journal, 0*(0). https://doi.org/10.1177/0032885512448604

Institute of Medicine (US) Committee on Ethical Considerations for Revisions to DHHS Regulations for Protection of Prisoners Involved in Research, Gostin, L. O., Vanchieri, C., & Pope, A. (Eds.). (2007). *Ethical considerations for research involving prisoners* (5th ed.). National Academies Press. https://www.ncbi.nlm.nih.gov/books/NBK19885/

Jones, L., Brookes, M., & Shuker, R. (2013). An exploration of cultural sensitivity: The experiences of offenders within a therapeutic community prison. *Race and Justice, 3*(2), 144–158. https://doi.org/10.1177/2153368713483324

Liu, K. A., & Dipietro Mager, N. A. (2016). Women's involvement in clinical trials: Historical perspective and future implications. *Pharmacy Practice (Granada), 14*(1), 0–0.

Moser, D. J., Arndt, S., Kanz, J. E., Benjamin, M. L., Bayless, J. D., Reese, R. L., Paulsen, J. S., & Flaum, M. A. (2004). Coercion and informed consent in research involving prisoners. *Comprehensive Psychiatry, 45*(1), 1–9. https://doi.org/10.1016/j.comppsych.2003.09.009

National Institute of Justice. (2012). National Institute of Justice Annual Report 2012 (NCJ 244249). U.S. Department of Justice, Office of Justice Programs. https://nij.ojp.gov/library/publications/national-institute-justice-annual-report-2012

Norcross, J. C., & Lambert, M. J. (2018). Psychotherapy relationships that work III. *Psychotherapy, 55*(4), 303–315. https://doi.org/10.1037/pst0000193

Oramas, J. E. (2017). Counseling ethics: Overview of challenges, responsibilities and recommended practices. *Journal of Multidisciplinary Research, 9*(3), 47–58.

Pack-Brown, S. P., Thomas, T. L., & Seymour, J. M. (2008). Infusing professional ethics in to counselor education programs: A multicultural/social justice perspective. *Journal of Counseling & Development, 86*(3), 296–302. https://doi.org/10.1002/j.1556-6678.2008.tb00512.x

Pennington, M., Patton, R., Ray, A., & Katafiasz, H. (2017). A brief report on the ethical and legal guides for technology use in marriage and family therapy. *Journal of Marital and Family Therapy, 43*(4), 733–742. https://doi.org/10.1111/jmft.12232

Peternelj-Taylor, C. (2004). An exploration of othering in forensic psychiatric and correctional nursing. *The Canadian Journal of Nursing Research = Revue canadienne de recherche en sciences infirmieres, 36*(4), 130–146.

Pont, J., Stöver, H., & Wolff, H. (2012). Dual loyalty in prison health care. *American Journal of Public Health, 102*(3), 475–480. https://doi.org/10.2105/AJPH.2011.300374

Pope, A. M. (2007). *Ethical considerations for research involving prisoners.* National Academies Press.

Simonds, V. W., Garroutte, E. M., & Buchwald, D. (2017). Health literacy and informed consent materials: designed for documentation, not comprehension of health research. *Journal of Health Communication, 22*(8), 682–691. https://doi.org/10.1080/10810730.2017.1341565

Tadros, E., Aguirre, N., Jensen, S., & Poehlmann-Tynan, J. (2021). COVID-19 inspired relational telemental health services for incarcerated individuals and their families. *Contemporary Family Therapy, 43*, 214–225. https://doi.org/10.1007/s10591-021-09578-6

Tadros, E., Fye, J. M., McCrone, C. L., & Finney, N. (2019). Incorporating multicultural couple and family therapy into incarcerated settings. *International Journal of Offender Therapy and Comparative Criminology, 63*(4), 641–658. https://doi.org/10.1177/0306624X18823442

Tadros, E., & Owens, D. (2021). Clinical implications for culturally informed counseling with incarcerated individuals. *The American Journal of Family Therapy, 49*(4), 344–355. https://doi.org/10.1080/01926187.2020.1813659

Tadros, E., Presley, S., & Guzman, Y. Z. (2023a). "Who are you really punishing?": Mothers' experiences with an incarcerated son. *Crime & Delinquency*. https://doi.org/10.1177/00111287221146544

Tadros, E., Salman, M., Ramadan, A., & Daifallah, N. (2023b). Community sadness: Clinical recommendations for working with grieving Arab American families. *The International Journal of Social Psychiatry, 69*(3), 602–612. https://doi.org/10.1177/00207640221124764

Tummala-Narra, P. (2015). Cultural competence as a core emphasis of psychoanalytic psychotherapy. *Psychodynamic Psychology, 32*(2), 275–292. https://doi.org/10.1037.a0034041

Van Westendorp, M., & Lierman, S. (2020). Walking the line: Balancing access to research and protecting prisoners. *Medical Law Review, 28*(1), 65–92. https://doi.org/10.1093/medlaw/fwy041

White, K. L., Jordens, C. F., & Kerridge, I. (2014). Contextualising professional ethics: The impact of the prison context on the practices and norms of health care practitioners. *Journal of Bioethical Inquiry, 11*(3), 333–345. https://doi.org/10.1007/s11673-014-9558-8

Chapter 9

Family Reunification

Romantic Partners Post-Release

Jeffrey Shewell and Eman Tadros

From time to time, many romantic relationships present with a variety of issues which lead to conflict. This is so, independent of the social location of its members or the population from which they come. It is an inevitability. However, it is because of the population within which they exist, that some relationships are more prone to conflict, in addition to facing issues notably unique to them. In cases where one member of the relationship was recently incarcerated and is now re-entering society, certain challenges are present that couples not of this population are less likely to encounter.

While issues of jealousy, feelings of inadequacy, and those related to expectations surrounding gender roles and responsibilities are not exclusive to romantic relationships within this population, these issues manifest in unique ways and may be particularly more pronounced for them. But in addition, issues which emerge from the threat of re-incarceration, a change in one partner's personality, a shift in familial roles, pent-up resentments, and barriers to employment, among many others, are novel to these romantic partnerships. The presence of these issues frequently leads to relationship dissolution. In fact, Turney (2015) names this outcome as one of the most common consequences of incarceration.

This chapter will explore the unique issues facing these couples, often leading to conflict and sometimes relationship dissolution. Existing protective factors against conflict will be explored and their inadequacy acknowledged. It will then review the scholarship that has previously made the case for therapeutic intervention as a necessity to overcome those inadequacies. It is worth noting that the majority of the literature focuses on incarcerated men and their non-incarcerated female partners, thus, this chapter will mirror that. Next, it will identify the role that marriage and family therapists (MFTs) can play in providing such interventions. This will include a review of research already performed on their efficacy. Lastly, two case studies will be presented demonstrating how this role may look, further supporting the claim that intervention by MFTs can positively impact relationship satisfaction among couples wherein one partner has been recently released from an incarceration facility.

DOI: 10.4324/9781003542940-9

That Was Then, This Is Now

During the incarceration period, non-incarcerated romantic partners are acutely aware of what the daily experience of their incarcerated partner entails. As discussed in previous chapters, correctional facilities are not conducive to the health and well-being of their individuals. Romantic partners are not naïve to this reality. In response, when communication between partners can occur, via face-to-face visits, phone calls, or letters, romantic partners often deliberately withhold the hardships they are encountering outside the walls of the correctional facility. Despite the facade, they are in fact affected by the incarceration just as much, but in their own ways, as their partner. Rather than disclose these hardships, a hopeful attitude which includes a feigned sense of optimism and encouragement is presented instead.

Not only do the non-incarcerated members of relationships shield their partners from distressing information, but the incarcerated also withhold from their partners many unpleasant truths related to their experience behind bars (DeHart et al., 2018). As a result of this unspoken agreement to limit conversation about stressful topics that may cause worry, concern, or disagreements between members of the relationship, the development of healthy communication techniques, coping strategies, and conflict resolution skills is neglected, natural progress in these areas is stunted, and any pre-existing presence of such interpersonal strengths is atrophied (Harman et al., 2007). While the implementation of such a strategy may be deliberate and arguably effective in easing the difficulties experienced by both partners during the incarceration period, the implications of this avoidance are typically overlooked and the repercussions become shockingly apparent only at the time of re-entry.

When the incarcerated individual is released, re-enters society, and is reunited with their romantic partner, the couple often finds that conflict and stressful topics can no longer be avoided. Issues that emerged during incarceration have built up, whether involving one partner or the other independent of each other or related to one another through the relationship they share together, and if the couple does not possess the necessary coping strategies or communication and conflict resolution skills required to address them, they almost assuredly give way to relationship distress (Comfort et al., 2018). Even if the couple does inherently possess well-developed skills and strategies in these domains, the compounding of issues over time, now befalling the couple all at once, rather than in piecemeal, may be overwhelming to the partnership and too much for the couple to address effectively and peaceably.

Another potentiality that may make conflict more pronounced, and specific to couples experiencing one of its member's recent release, is the "behavioral deep freeze", when an incarcerated individual's "set of outside-world behaviors are stored until his release" (Zamble & Porporino, 1990, p.62). The behaviors that led to an individual becoming incarcerated, they explain, lay dormant, constrained by the policies of the correctional facility, but are never addressed in such a way as to alter or overcome them. At the time of re-entry, the latent behaviors "unfreeze", as the individual is no longer subject to the rules and policies of the correctional facility that restricted them or kept them contained, and the individual returns to the outside world no more socially or behaviorally developed than when they left it (Zamble & Porporino, 1990).

Harman et al. (2007) explained through their contrasting of the coping strategies and communication skills of the incarcerated individual, which have been stunted and remain the same as they were at the time of incarceration, with those of their partner, who, having changed and grown while living freely in the outside world, has had the opportunity to better hone and develop their utilization of these skills and strategies. Whereas the couple may have had a congruent way of navigating conflict prior to incarceration, following the incarcerated partner's release, the couple may now find that their respective approaches to addressing conflict are incompatible, presenting increased difficulties between the two in navigating whatever personal or relationship issues that may have emerged during incarceration, as well as those that arose only at the time of re-entry.

It is no wonder that some couples report being happier in their relationship during incarceration than during the re-entry period (Comfort et al., 2018). Relationships affected by the incarceration of one of its members exist amidst extraordinary circumstances, compelling both partners to put on their best face and to willingly set aside any conflictual topics, deliberately omitting them from conversation in the interest of sustaining one another's mental and emotional well-being. Disruptively and abruptly, however, at the time of re-entry, this facade of placating optimism and of a well-meaning, although hollow, sense of hopefulness is shattered, and the stunted growth of the incarcerated individual's interpersonal skills becomes apparent. Such a deficit in their development becomes only more apparent when contrasted with the assumed strengthening of such skills by their partner, who has had just as much time outside of bars, as their partner did behind them, to develop these skills through a multitude of varying interactions, relationships, and experiences. Such relational dissonance causes a collision at the time of re-entry, as the compounding of issues avoided during incarceration now suddenly becomes unavoidable, leaving couples ill-prepared to navigate the face-to-face encounter with their new reality.

Romantic partners navigating re-entry may look back upon the incarceration period as one during which the relationship was marked less by conflict and dissatisfaction, and more by teamwork, solidarity, and shared optimism. Paradoxically, self-reports made by both partners indicate that the presence of relationship happiness, relationship quality, and the level of supportiveness, significantly decreases in the period following the man's release from a correctional facility (Turney, 2015). This trend can be attributed not only to the couple's inability to avoid unaddressed issues which emerged during the incarceration period, but also to the unanticipated issues that commonly arise exclusively at the time of re-entry, issues which this chapter will now explore (Comfort et al., 2018).

Unmet Expectations in the Aftermath of Incarceration

An individual's incarceration can have significant impacts on the loved ones and family members who had previously relied upon them for financial support. Not only do non-incarcerated partners, oftentimes sharing children with the incarcerated individual, frequently lose an entire income source and struggle adapting to functioning as a single parent as a result of their loved one's incarceration, but they also become more financially burdened by new expenses. Non-incarcerated romantic partners eagerly anticipate their loved one's release with the expectation that this event will alleviate the additional financial burden they have shouldered for the duration of their loved one's sentence. No longer must they shoulder the cost of supporting their loved one in prison, but in fact, they now instead will have a second source of income to support the household and any potential children they might share together. However, this optimistic anticipation is frequently met with disappointment and unmet expectations when said loved one is released because, although the non-incarcerated partner no longer must cover communication and commissary costs, the financial support they previously received from their loved one prior to incarceration does not necessarily return just because their partner has been released. Instead, it is frequently the case that a formerly incarcerated individual remains dependent on their romantic partner to meet their own basic needs, unable to offer anything in the way of financial support as a result of the barriers to employment experienced by former convicts (Harman et al., 2007).

The non-incarcerated person hopes that their partner's release will provide them with much-needed relief from the heavy financial and emotional burden that their incarceration had placed on them. However, released individuals often struggle to find employment and meet household expectations, generating feelings of disappointment, frustration, and resentment within their partner, and oftentimes leading to conflict (Comfort et al., 2018). The anticipated "return to normalcy" or a better "new normal" often falls short, increasing the partner's disappointment.

As a result, some formerly incarcerated men report placing a greater level of importance on finding a job and achieving a sense of stability, financial or otherwise, than focusing on their relationship. According to Comfort et al. (2018), this mentality "left their relationships in limbo [at the time of reentry], with uncertainty about whether or not the partnership would eventually become a focal point again" (p.195). These men believe that only once they have established this stability, can they then begin focusing on their relationship and any existing issues with their romantic partner, whether having emerged as a result of their incarceration and their now recent release, or otherwise (Harman et al., 2007).

Prior to incarceration, men who engaged in recurring behaviors, infidelity, substance use, or neglected parental responsibilities, put strain on their partners, thus contributing to high levels of relationship distress. Throughout the incarceration period, however, incarcerated men sometimes reflect on their actions and express to their partner a desire to change, increasing the level of hopefulness that their partner has for their release (Turney, 2015). However, upon release, some men may fail to maintain the sense of dedication to living a reformed life they had previously expressed while incarcerated, shattering the positive expectations their partners had for them. Consequently, many women become fearful that their partner's inability to follow through on these commitments will lead to re-incarceration; a fearfulness that can foster further discord in the relationship (Turney, 2015).

Even in instances where there is reform after release, some women still report struggling to adjust to their return. Having needed to adapt to their partner's absence, they often have developed a sense of independence and resourcefulness that they found empowering. They may have needed only to care for themselves and any children within the household while their partner was incarcerated. Upon his release, the routines that she had developed to provide for herself, and her children are disrupted, as she now needs to account for and take into consideration another adult as well, whom, due to barriers to employment, she may now become financially responsible for (Comfort et al., 2018).

Feelings of Inadequacy, Emotional Withdrawal, and the Threat of Re-incarceration

Previously incarcerated men shared with researchers a strong desire to reestablish themselves post-release, while expressing sentiments that implied doing so was predicated on successfully obtaining employment (Comfort et al., 2018). In pursuit of this goal, however, and to their dismay, they reported encountering major barriers all stemming from their previous involvement with the criminal justice system. It was subsequently made apparent that securing a reliable and independently earned source of income was desirable not only because it would serve the function of meeting one's family's material needs, but it would also help previously incarcerated and recently released men secure the degree of self-sustainability and stability necessary for them to maintain the sense of self-worth, self-confidence, autonomy, and self-esteem that would effectively overcome many of the soon to be explored challenges couples face at the time of re-entry.

Unfortunately, because all has been predicated upon a recently released person's ability to secure employment, which is particularly challenging for them given their criminal background, men develop feelings of inadequacy in response to, not only their inability to support their family, but also because of their very dependence on their family for survival. Feelings of both shame and guilt can emerge as a result (Comfort et al., 2018). The reckoning they face with their new reality, which is accompanied by high levels of emotional discomfort and deep feelings of inadequacy, may cause these men to withdraw or isolate from their partners and family, creating physical and emotional distance, for the purpose of psychological self-preservation, carried out through acts of avoidance (Harman et al., 2007).

Interviews with female partners of incarcerated men indicate that this guilt and shame is not merely a result of men's own internalized feelings of inadequacy but has some basis in their immediate realities (Harman et al., 2007). Some of the women interviewed explicitly vocalized feelings of anger directed at their partner for the loss of income, the loss of child support, and the loss of a second parent to assist with child rearing, all a result of their incarceration. One woman in particular expressed frustration specifically *because* her incarcerated partner could not fulfill the traditional male role of provider she expected him to, but instead, felt as though it was now expected of her to take on this role, which stood in stark contrast to her personal values, requiring her to provide for him, through the provision of commissary payments and by covering the cost of collect calls.

So, although this identity of "provider" may have been previously internalized by these men independent of external influences, the frustration and disappointment, certainly not ill-placed, expressed by their partners toward them, has only further served to generate a great deal of inner turmoil for men recently released from incarceration. In concordance with these interviews, men who were interviewed post-release reported that pressure put on them by their partner to become financially stable, in the face of their earnest efforts to do so, and amidst the insurmountable barriers rendering such efforts futile, only served to intensify feelings of inadequacy (Harman et al., 2007).

The desire to escape these unpleasant emotions can lead some men simply to prioritize socializing with friends over spending time with or focusing on their families, while in other cases, recently released men are inclined to engage in much riskier behaviors. This physical and emotional absence can cause their partners to fear that they are returning to criminal behaviors or resorting to drug use, which in many cases is true. Many men do feel inclined and in fact do return to drug dealing or other criminal behaviors to once again begin providing for their family financially. Simultaneously, this also occurs for more personal reasons, such actions being taken as a means to resolve their own feelings of guilt, shame, and inadequacy, feelings which they find incredibly uncomfortable to experience (Harman et al., 2007).

These actions, when carried out by men, instill a substantiated, reasonable fear within their female partners, as they face the very real possibility that their partner may become re-incarcerated. Consequently, the prospect of such a possibility becoming reality often prevents them from fully engaging in their romantic relationship or from investing time, energy, and emotion into strengthening their bond. Such fear, as self-reported by these women, serves as a barrier to intimacy and dampens the desire to reestablish their romantic connection (Harman et al., 2007). The disengagement of women from their romantic relationships, carried out as an act of self-preservation inspired by the fear they feel in response to the very plausible scenario that their partner might become re-incarcerated, although reasonable, understandable, and substantiated by the reality of experience, introduces the unfortunate consequence of further isolating their recently released male partner. Already struggling with feelings of inadequacy, guilt, and shame, he is now suffering from an experience of isolation and alienation. The negative emotional state already present at the time of the initial reengagement in his primary intimate relationship is further exacerbated.

These factors compound and, although inadvertently, the two partners behave in ways that, despite being out of self-preservation, bring further distress to the relationship, not only increasing the likelihood of dissolution, but increasing the likelihood of the male partner's return to criminal behavior and increasing the likelihood of recidivism and re-incarceration. The female partner, again, self-preserves and withdraws in response to this fear, creating and solidifying a self-sustaining and self-perpetuating cycle that has the potential to continue indefinitely and, unfortunately, often precipitates disastrous results.

Is This the Same Person I Fell in Love with?

Harman et al. (2007) interviewed formerly incarcerated men and non-incarcerated female partners to understand the experience of reuniting with their loved ones after an extended separation. "Most participants", they found, "reported feeling like very different people after their separation" and as though they needed to "get to know each other all over again" (p.801). Respondents frequently expressed the sentiment that they felt as though they no longer knew their partner or that the reunion experienced at the time of re-entry ushered in the beginnings of a brand new relationship that could only survive if the couple returned to the start, rebuilding the relationship from the bottom up as if they had just met each other for the first time (Harman et al., 2007). The decision to do so, however, is a perilous one, and is not always made, out of fear and apprehension rooted in a variety of reasons and which this chapter just previously explored.

Turney (2015) notes that not only does the resulting separation caused by incarceration create a sense of unfamiliarity between partners at the time of release, but the incarceration itself can have significant effects on the personality and constitution of the incarcerated partner. The quality of a person's mental health can be seriously diminished because of incarceration as they adjust to the stressors that confinement brings with it. Upon release, this diminishment remains present, and the effects of the confinement may be long-lasting, reducing the quality of communication and the intimacy experienced between romantic partners.

Articles have documented that individuals who are incarcerated in correctional facilities develop trauma-based symptoms consistent with post-traumatic stress disorder, including depression, hyper-vigilance, anxiety, isolation, and emotional numbing (Charles et al., 2019). The emergence of these symptoms occurs within this population at a rate 2–10 times higher than among non-incarcerated members of society, and their prevalence among this population ranges from somewhere between 4% and 21%. And this reality is not lost on the female partners of formerly incarcerated men. Harman et al. (2007) reported that some women specifically remarked on changes in personality they observed in their partner upon re-entry, particularly their unusual level of quietness, which took months for them to overcome. Adapting to, understanding, and ultimately accepting the negative effects that incarceration has had on one's partner's mental health can be challenging.

In addition to the detrimental effect life behind bars can have on an individual's mental health, from which relationship distress emerges as an indirect consequence, incarceration may also be accompanied by direct consequences impacting interpersonal relations themselves, in the form of unhealthy and maladaptive methods through which post-release individuals address conflict in their romantic partnerships. Hairston and Oliver (2006) found that female partners of incarcerated men feared that the development of a "prison mentality" would be detrimental to the men's ability to maintain healthy relationships post-release. In elaboration, Stansfield et al. (2020) suggest that correctional facilities create a culture which necessitates outward displays of bravado by incarcerates and the embracing of hyper-masculine qualities such as toughness and aggressiveness as a means of survival, resulting in an inability once released to navigate conflict in ways that are appropriate and culturally acceptable by the standards aspired to by free society. In conclusion, they present the possibility that conflict and violence emerge between recently incarcerated individuals and their partners not solely due to the separation from one another they had to endure, noting that the vastly different experiences of the partners during the incarceration period have created an incongruence on a psychological level which may be just as much responsible.

The "tools" that an individual needs to "survive" in a correctional facility are vastly different from the tools needed to maintain a healthy romantic relationship on the outside. Concerns exist that, once released, formerly incarcerated men may retain the utilization of such maladaptive tools in the interpersonal relationships in which they engage after they have been released and have re-entered society, leading to, at best, relationship discord, and at worst, intimate partner violence. This important and very serious topic will be considered later.

Distance Makes the Heart Grow... Fonder?

If "distance makes the heart grow fonder", as the saying goes, then incarceration can make jealousy and mistrust grow. Both men and women believe that the base level of anxiety experienced by many men due to concerns about their partner's fidelity is intensified by incarceration. This elevation is attributed to physical separation, difficulties in or even a complete inability to contact or communicate with one another, and a general sense of powerlessness that incarceration naturally provokes. On this topic, women have reported that when contact and communication had occurred, this anxiety manifested in ways that included their incarcerated partner questioning them about their whereabouts or making accusations about their involvement with other men (Comfort et al., 2018).

These feelings of jealousy can be further fueled by rumors that emerge and are shared with the incarcerated partner by community members, friends, or family members on the outside, with whom they are in contact (Comfort et al., 2018). This outside influence on the prominence of jealousy and concerns about infidelity is substantiated by complementary research wherein non-incarcerated women reported feeling as though they were "under constant surveillance from family, friends, and their communities", making them apprehensive to even "socialize or seek support", out of "fear that infidelity rumors would lead back to their [incarcerated] partners" (Harman et al., 2007, p.800).

This expectation of fidelity, and an inability while incarcerated to know with certainty whether a romantic partner is in fact remaining faithful, leads to suspicions and accusations. But while there is very little if anything the incarcerated partner can do to address these concerns at the time, such anxieties and insecurities could give way to conflict between couples post-release, once the incarcerated partner regains a level of power and control that they had been lacking while away. And although interviewed women of incarcerated male partners reported remaining loyal to them for the duration of their sentence, citing that functioning as single parents and adapting to subsisting on a single income was too overwhelming and preoccupying for them to even think about sex or other men, many held the belief that their incarcerated partners would not remain faithful themselves were their situations reversed (Harman et al., 2007).

While incarcerated individuals are inclined to be faithful to their partners, for the obvious reason that they may experience limited opportunities to engage in infidelity, upon release, a double-standard sometimes emerges, wherein the previously jealous and suspicious partner begins themself to engage in romantic or sexual relationships outside their primary partnership. Women of formerly incarcerated men have reported that upon re-entry, their partners engaged in multiple romantic and/or sexual relationships with other women, leading them to end the relationship altogether. And while research has shown that few men self-report not remaining exclusive to their partners post-release, others do admit to it. In those instances, one reason given revealed an overall feeling of entitlement expressed by the male partner, a feeling possessed as a result of having been deprived of so much while incarcerated. Research found that collectively, men expressed a desire to take advantage of their newly granted freedom in such a way that prioritized their own wants and wishes over those of others, an outlook incompatible with the requirements serious and committed relationships frequently demand (Comfort et al., 2018).

Existing Protective Factors Against Conflict Post-Release

The issues just explored, although widespread, do not lead to conflict or relationship dissolution in all instances. The presence of certain factors has been quantitatively linked to a decrease in the frequency of such outcomes. Such factors include the length of the relationship prior to the incarceration period and the sharing and coparenting of at least one child together. The belief in being bonded with one's partner after having been in a relationship for many years may lead to a belief that anything, including separation by incarceration, can be overcome. The duration of the relationship prior to incarceration and the belief in the importance of maintaining the relationship for the sake of shared children have both been qualitatively studied and reported as influencing the likelihood that couples will remain together post-release (Comfort et al., 2018).

Furthermore, previous studies have shown an indirect correlation between the frequency of in-person family visits and the presence of family conflict post-release. And although face-to-face interactions have been demonstrated to be most effective in reducing the likelihood of family conflict during the re-entry period, it has also been demonstrated that communication of any kind, even when by telephone or written letters, serves as a protective factor against post-release family conflict (Stansfield et al., 2020). Regular communication with loved ones through the duration of one's incarceration serves as an anchor, grounding an incarcerated individual's experience to the world outside of prison and with those they share a connection, reminding them of the temporality of their current situation and preparing them for a return to the world that they previously knew but had to leave behind.

However, it is not always the case that couples have been together for an extended period prior to incarceration, nor is it always so that the couple shares children together. It is also important to acknowledge that even when these factors are present, they do not guarantee that conflict won't still arise. And although regular communication between family members and the incarcerated population has been highly documented as an effective deterrent against post-release familial conflict, this deterrent is demonstrably insufficient for a variety of reasons:

1 Barriers to regular face-to-face visits are many in number. Having been previously discussed in an earlier chapter, revisiting such barriers reminds us that they include: the proximity of the prison to a family's residence, lack of reliable transportation, limited finances which prevent travel and deter family members from missing work, overly strict and stringent dress code requirements, and finally the inaccessibility of childcare and restrictions to child needs during the duration of the visit. High cost of telephone calls makes even this form of communication difficult for some families (Comfort et al., 2005).
2 Despite the positive effect of regular family contact during the incarceration period, post-release family conflict is often still present, even when such contact occurred with a moderate degree of consistency (Stansfield et al., 2020). The reported reduction of conflict due to regular family contact is insufficient to not still demand further interventions.
3 Although regular family contact decreases the level of conflict during the re-entry period, rates of family violence appear to be unaffected by this factor post-release (Stansfield et al., 2020). Family violence among those affected by incarceration deserves specific attention.

Understanding the Relationship between Family Violence and Incarceration

Stansfield et al. (2020) examined 1,282 incarcerated men, interviewing them pre-release and up to three times within 15 months after release. The study found that family contact during incarceration reduced post-release family conflict but did not impact the occurrence of family violence after re-entry. Studies have demonstrated a decrease in the presence of family violence post-release compared to the pre-release period; however, based on reports made by study participants, it's been revealed that the presence of conflict resolution skills was more likely responsible for this decrease than regular family contact was (McKay et al., 2018). This further demonstrates the importance that therapeutic interventions occur at the point of re-entry, as this would provide opportunities for conflict resolution skills to become more fully developed.

Although regular family contact is not correlated with family violence post-release, substance use is positively correlated with the presence of intimate partner violence (IPV) (Cafferky et al., 2018). Stansfield et al. (2020) have replicated these findings. Given that recently released men experience a variety of challenges and stressors, as this chapter has discussed, and therefore may be inclined to begin using substances again, despite having remained substance free for the duration of their sentence, the potential for relapse is high and serves as a risk factor for post-release IPV. The need for therapeutic interventions upon re-entry is therefore made further apparent due to this reality.

Despite a decrease in the presence of family violence pre- and post-release, research has concluded that its presence still remains higher among families affected by incarceration than those who are not, both prior to incarceration and following re-entry (Stansfield et al., 2020). Therapeutic interventions at the time of re-entry would therefore provide an opportunity to address this issue within a population in which its presence is more prevalent, independent of any factors that may have already decreased the likelihood that it will in fact occur.

Only a nominal amount of research has been conducted on the impact of MFTs in improving relationship quality between partners post-release. In fact, there exists limited research exploring the impact systemic therapeutic interventions may have on any familial relationships during this period, not just limited to romantic partnerships. Negash et al. (2022) note this while also identifying the multitude of barriers to such research being conducted, including: cultural and community stigma surrounding mental health and therapeutic services, a lack of cultural awareness and competency on the part of therapists, difficulties in logistically planning for relevant family members to be present, internalized stigmas possessed by post-release men about appearing weak or vulnerable, among many others.

Despite the limited research on the impact of MFTs, or comparable interventions, on the well-being of romantic partnerships post-release, there does exist a valuable body of literature on the positive impact of their involvement during the incarceration period. This section will explore this literature and then extrapolate from it, as a means to demonstrate how such involvement could be equally beneficial during the post-release period. Finally, a proposal for MFT involvement will be illustrated through, and the efficacy of such involvement substantiated by, the presentation of two case examples depicting the successful interventions of MFTs in treating couples as they navigate the post-release period. These illustrations are fictional representations, despite this, the cases are informed by the literature reviewed, which included: an exploration of issues which occur frequently and are commonly experienced by couples during the post-release period, evidence of a need, and a precedence of scholarly awareness of the need, for services to address these issues, as well as an examination of MFT involvement and its proven efficacy in treating couples during the incarceration period.

A study by Jalali and colleagues (2017) in Iran to determine whether the use of Solution-Focused Brief Couples Therapy had any positive impact on the relationship quality reported by currently incarcerated men and their wives was published. Although sessions were not conducted by MFTs, SFBCT is a therapeutic approach commonly utilized by MFTs in the United States, and the therapists participating in the study did possess the appropriate credentials recognized by their country's overseeing body. Thus, the implications of the research findings are nonetheless highly relevant and valuable to this chapter's purpose.

The study consisted of 50 men, then incarcerated at Mashhad Central Prison in Mashhad, Iran, and their non-incarcerated wives, with all couples volunteering for the study and being selected from a total of 120 applicants after being screened and deemed to have met the studies eligibility requirements. The couples were divided into two groups of 25, with the experimental group receiving six sessions of SFBCT and the control group receiving none. Due to limitations pre-existing within the prison's mode of operation, only two of the six sessions were carried out with both partners present together, the other four sessions were conducted with each partner separately. The collection of data involved participants completing a 35-item assessment on a 5-point Likert scale which was divided into 4 subscales measuring the presence of "Marital Satisfaction", "Communication", "Conflict Resolution", and "Idealistic Distortion". Assessments were given prior to the first session and then again after the final session.

The results of the study showed a markedly pronounced difference in outcomes between the experimental and control group, with the experimental group reporting a significant improvement across participants in marital satisfaction, communication, and "conflict resolution", and a significant decrease in the presence of idealistic distortion. In contrast, changes in the control group's pre- and post-assessment ratings were statistically negligible. These results contribute to the ever-blooming recognition among therapists, scholars, and academics that therapeutic interventions–particularly those which understand individuals' experiences to be inseparable from their relationships with others–can improve the quality of life among both incarcerated men and their partners.

MFTs practicing within the U.S. have also published literature summarizing their experiences working with incarcerated individuals and their partners prior to re-entry. Tadros and Smithee (2022) demonstrated the positive impact that MFTs could have on the relationship quality of partners experiencing the deleterious effects of incarceration through a case study involving a lesbian couple who received therapy while one partner was still serving out their sentence. In this case study, therapy was provided through the utilization of the Tadros Theory of Change, an integrative approach to couples and family therapy which roots itself in Minuchin's (1974) structural family therapy, while also incorporating elements prominent within the narrative as well as solution-focused approaches (Tadros, 2019).

The Tadros Theory of Change (2019) is a systemic theory that seeks to empower clients to define goals for themselves, for the purpose of overcoming problems they have identified within their lives or relationships. This collaborative, client-driven method is derived from the solution-focused approach proven to be effective in helping to address presenting issues brought by clients to the therapy room in the most expedient and efficacious way. Unique to the Tadros approach however, is the cultural humility inherent within it and upon which the theory is reliant, in order to recognize that, as a highly marginalized and consistently overlooked population, those affected by incarceration may suffer from a sense of feeling their voice is not heard, that their future is unclear, and that hope is lost. Therapists may struggle to fully grasp this reality to the extent necessary to effectively facilitate the empowerment required for clients to confidently identify problems, define goals, and seek solutions. Clients may lack confidence from the lack of autonomy experienced, and subsequently internalized, after spending time surviving within a correctional facility (Tadros, 2021). The Tadros Theory of Change recognizes the existing limitations of the therapist, the understated but omnipresent apprehensions of the client, and reconciles the two, effectively and successfully bridging the gap.

In pursuit of achieving the goals identified by the client, in the solution-focused tradition, techniques found within the structural approach assist clients in identifying, setting, and respecting healthy boundaries. Narrative theory is integral through its effectiveness at helping incarcerated clients challenge the stories they find themselves living out, through assisting them in altering their language, in order that they can create new stories for themselves, reshaping their values, their self-identity, and the way they understand their circumstances (Tadros, 2021).

In a case study by Tadros and Smithee (2022), in which the Tadros Theory of Change was utilized, a lesbian couple received therapy at the facility where one partner was serving a minimum two-year sentence for illegal possession of narcotics. Both partners had previously attained sobriety together, meeting in a 12-step group, and subsequently maintained years of sobriety while in romantic partnership with one another, up until the recent relapse, which eventually led to the incarceration. Therapy was sought by the couple in hopes that it could assist them in adjusting to the changes in the nature of the relationship due to the incarceration, in helping to cope with the stressors that had subsequently arisen, and due to sexual dissatisfaction, which had emerged months before the incarceration period began. Ultimately, the couple sought to avoid relationship dissolution (Tadros & Smithee, 2022).

The therapist applied the structural technique of joining with the couple to develop a strong therapeutic alliance with clients whose experience is unique from much of the population, given that one is incarcerated and that they are in a lesbian relationship. Joining helped the therapist to affirm and validate the clients' experience and helped the clients feel understood and as though they could trust and open up to the therapist. Furthermore, in the structural tradition, the therapist reframed the identified problem of one partner's low-sex drive to change the couple's focus, broaden perspectives on their situation, and reduce blame. In doing so, the situation was presented as being more relational in nature, rather than individual, in a way that systems theory, implemented by MFTs, can do arguably more successfully than approaches which view problems as being solely individualistic in nature (Tadros & Smithee, 2022).

It was also found that in addition to sexual dissatisfaction, one partner felt as though the other was ashamed of her, compounded by her partner's experiences within her family of origin, having been raised in a family less tolerant toward the LGBTQ+ community. Much unresolved and underattended to anger was present as a result of this perceived shame. This revelation was made recognizable through the efforts of the therapist in seeking input from both partners as to what they viewed the problem within their relationship to be. It was found that the identified problems, as identified by both clients, were very much connected with one another and could not have been addressed in isolation. Narrative techniques were utilized to create a shared story for the couple, successfully overcoming barriers to connection that they had been experiencing and to assist in understanding one another more fairly and with greater acceptance. This included understanding the role that shame, and religion can play in one's social location as a woman in a romantic lesbian relationship, as well as the unique experience of a lesbian within a correctional facility (Tadros & Smithee, 2022).

This new mutual understanding for one another created a sense of hopefulness and willingness necessary to make changes, allowing for solution-focused techniques to be successful in their execution. The therapist subsequently guided the couple as they came up with unique and creative, concrete ways that they could develop and maintain a level of intimacy to the greatest extent that their separation would permit. With a new understanding of the problems facing their relationship, and a new understanding of one another, the clients successfully completed therapy, and services were terminated (Tadros & Smithee, 2022).

Although this example involves a romantic couple receiving therapy while one partner is currently incarcerated, rather than one in which therapy is provided during the post-release period, it does demonstrate several things relevant to achieving this chapter's aims. Utilizing a systems approach, a MFT was able to successfully assist a romantic couple navigate and overcome the issues threatening their relationship. Although some of the problems facing this couple would not be uncommon in couples unaffected by incarceration, in this instance, incarceration intensified and complicated these problems, while also introducing situations and experiences unique to this population. And despite services being provided prior to release, it has already been demonstrated that, although different in scope in many ways, the problems that emerge post-release are also a direct result of the incarceration experience.

With these considerations, it is not without substantiation to draw the conclusion that, if couples therapy can be effective at preventing relationship dissolution due to issues unique to the incarceration period, then such intervention can be effective in preventing this outcome similarly when used to address issues unique to the post-release period. In both cases, incarceration plays an enormous role in contributing to presenting problems experienced by romantic partners, and MFTs can play a vital role in assisting these couples in overcoming them.

Case Example 1

Marcus is a 36-year-old, African American male who has recently been released from federal prison after serving 9 years for drug trafficking and criminal possession of an unlicensed firearm. His romantic partner of 12 years, Lisa (32 years old, African American, female), chose to maintain their relationship for the duration of his sentence, supporting him financially during his incarceration, visiting him as frequently as possible, while also serving as the sole provider and caregiver to their two children (now aged 11 and 10). Lisa relied heavily on her parents for support during Marcus' incarceration and worked multiple part-time jobs supplemented by public assistance to meet the needs of her and the couple's children.

Upon release, Marcus felt an obligation to fulfill the traditional paternalistic, male gender role by providing for both his partner and his children. Marcus experienced barriers to fulfilling this role as a result of difficulties in obtaining employment due to his status as a felon. Meanwhile, having been the sole source of income for the family for those nine years, Lisa had experienced great hardship ensuring that all four members of the family's needs were met. Meanwhile, she grew to resent Marcus for the financial costs specifically associated with his incarceration, which included pricey collect calls, commissary payments, and expenses incurred from traveling over an hour for face-to-face visits, as well as the strain it placed on her parents in terms of assistance in child-rearing and childcare.

Lisa held high expectations for Marcus' release, anticipating that with it she would experience an alleviation of the weight of hardships she had shouldered for the family as a consequence of his incarceration. Lisa assumed without question that Marcus would resume his place in the family as financial provider and reclaim the position of head of household, guardian, father, and leader. She expected Marcus to return from prison motivated and determined to "right the wrongs", repair the damage, and solve the problems facing his family which Lisa attributed to his incarceration.

Although Marcus was unaware of these expectations, Lisa having never communicated them to him, Marcus already possessed almost identical expectations for himself, having internalized the very same role for himself that Lisa had attributed to him in her mind. However, when Marcus found it difficult to alleviate the financial hardship Lisa had been experiencing due to his status as a felon, he began to experience feelings of inadequacy and shame. Co-occurring with this experience, feelings of disappointment in Marcus' inability to meet her expectations began to arise in Lisa. Eventually, unaware of the shame and highly critical self-image Marcus was becoming afflicted by, Lisa began to communicate her disappointment in Marcus, at first subtly in passing, through sarcasm or thinly veiled insults disguised as jokes (for example, commenting after his release on how she went from having only two mouths to feed to now three), and eventually directly and emphatically (for example, telling him how she struggled to make ends meet while he was incarcerated and how, without him working, he might as well still be locked up). The hope of relief from hardship that carried her through the worst of his incarceration no longer alleviated the stress and suffering she experienced, and all of the bottled-up resentment was released indiscriminately. Already feeling emasculated, but unbeknownst to Lisa, Marcus' shame and guilt became overwhelming and he became emotionally withdrawn and physically absent. Unfortunately, this only served to increase the conflict.

Marcus considers returning to criminal behaviors to provide for his family, to alleviate the stress that Lisa is experiencing, to save their relationship by assuming the role of primary provider, and to address his own feelings of inadequacy as being dependent on his romantic partner. Marcus also feels a pull to avoid Lisa and his children all together, for the purpose of escapism and emotional self-preservation. The stress Marcus feels at home inclines him instead to want to spend time with old friends, ignore his responsibilities to his family, and protect himself emotionally.

The more Marcus pulls away from the family, as an act of self-preservation, to save himself from his feelings of inadequacy as a provider, the more Lisa becomes fearful not only that he has become unwilling to step into the role she expects of him, but that he will become incapable of doing so, because he has already, or will soon, become involved in criminal behaviors. Lisa is conflicted because she misses the life they had before he was incarcerated, and the financial stability they enjoyed, but also knows that if he reoffends, he will certainly become re-incarcerated. Meanwhile, Marcus experiences a similar internal struggle over what actions he should take. Lisa begins to withdraw herself, ambivalent now about her feelings, which Marcus notices. Confused by this, Marcus fears that Lisa has given up on him. He begins to experience a sense of urgency to take some form of action to provide for his family, to prove to himself and to Lisa that he is capable.

Given the demonstrated efficacy of the Tadros Theory of Change in assisting traditionally marginalized populations affected by incarceration, as was explored in the previous section (sexually minoritized couple), the therapist who would be working with Marcus and Lisa (racially minoritized couple) wished to see if this approach could be equally effective when utilized, not during the incarceration period, but instead, after Marcus had been released.

In fidelity to the Tadros Theory, the therapist placed strong emphasis in the early sessions on developing a therapeutic alliance with the couple adequate in strength to overcome any socio-economic or cultural barriers that might exist as a result of the therapist not belonging to the African-American community. This was made more achievable through the therapist's reliance on the technique of joining, which involved acknowledging their own limitations on understanding the African-American experience having knowledge of it only through hearing the accounts shared with them by members of this community, what they had read and studied on their own, and through working closely with members of this community in a professional capacity in the past (Tadros & Smithee, 2022).

The therapist shared that they were aware that persons of color are disproportionately subjected to interactions with the police, are disproportionately affected by mass incarceration in the United States, and on average receive longer sentences than Caucasian Americans for similar convictions. The therapist also acknowledged that economic opportunities are less available to persons of color, especially those residing in urban settings. Despite this awareness brought with them to the therapy room, the therapist expressed a desire to hear Marcus and Lisa share their experiences as individual persons, regardless of how similar or unlike they may be to the therapist's generalized knowledge on the experience of African-Americans.

The therapist then proceeded to ask both Marcus and Lisa individually what they identified as the problem in their relationship which ultimately brought them to therapy. Marcus shared that he is worried Lisa has given up on him and is going to leave him because he can't provide for his family. He shared that he "hates himself" for not being able to take care of them the way he wants to and knows he should. Lisa shared that she doesn't want the family torn apart, that she hasn't even considered leaving Marcus, that it would solve nothing, but is disappointed that he hasn't "stepped up" the way she expected him to after he returned home.

Adhering to the Tadros Theory's blending of structural and solution-focused approaches, the therapist paid appropriate attention to the content provided by the clients, presenting itself in the form of pervasive themes within their story such as traditional gender roles, shame, resentment, expectations, the African American identity, financial hardship, and inadequate communication skills while also encouraging the couple to remain future-oriented and positively minded as they collaboratively identified goals for therapy and considered what possible solutions might look like. In doing so, the therapist fostered an environment in which both Marcus and Lisa began to speak more broadly about their histories both independent of one another and once they became a couple. The therapist sought to incorporate the narrative elements relied upon by the Tadros Theory to better understand them as clients as well as to create an opportunity for them to better understand one another as partners. The eventual rewriting of their story would be tethered to the solutions they will have collaboratively identified for themselves as a couple. Both partners spoke independently of one another about their own perspectives on and understanding of expected gender roles within a family. Neither account deviated significantly from the others. However, it was Marcus' recounting of his position within his family of origin, and of how he found himself in that position, that was the most revealing, providing a rich narrative linking his past to his present.

Growing up, Marcus shared that he was the oldest of four children. He had some early memories of his father which he described positively but quickly explained how by the time he was nearing age 9 or 10, he recalls only seeing his father sporadically and infrequently. Marcus shared that his dad wanted him and his younger siblings to like him when he would appear in their lives unannounced, temporarily, after extended periods of absence, but that he did not respect him and didn't play along with his games. Marcus shared that instead, he saw his mom struggling to provide for him and his younger siblings and grew to hate his father for, as he saw it, being responsible for the difficulties that his mother was facing. Marcus shared that he wasn't exactly sure where the belief came from, but he remembers always believing that it was the man's job to provide for his children and their mother, whether they were together or not, because if the mother is struggling, then the children are struggling. Marcus doesn't remember anyone explicitly telling him that he needed to step up and assume the role of provider in the home in his father's absence, but as the oldest, he felt it was his duty to do so.

Marcus explained that he was eventually taken under the wing of a few older teenagers who helped him out by fronting him some weed so he could start to make a little bit of money and establish a clientele. Not long after, Marcus had accumulated enough money that he didn't have to rely on the favors of others, and he became very motivated and self-driven. Marcus used the money to help make sure that his family had what they needed, even though they still had to go without a lot of the time. Over the years, Marcus got deeper into drug dealing until he was trafficking fairly large quantities of much harder drugs, necessitating with it the ability to protect himself and his business through the possession of firearms.

Lisa's narrative overlapped with Marcus' at this point, recalling that when she met him, she felt safe and provided for. She as well had experienced poverty growing up and the sense of security that she believed Marcus could provide was attractive to her, noting that she did actually fall in love with him too as a person, that it was not just about his ability to provide for her materially. Their stories remained parallel up until Marcus' incarceration. They had two children together and believed that nothing could go wrong. Marcus' unexpected arrest and subsequent sentence turned their lives upside down.

From both of their accounts, the therapist gathered that for the first few years of Marcus' incarceration, the couple held firmly to their bond and their shared determination to get through this together. However, as the years went on, while Marcus continued to trust in this bond and the assurance that Lisa was steadfast in her commitment to their partnership, Lisa revealed that she became overwhelmed by the hardships she experienced as a single mother struggling to provide for her family financially (paying rent, affording groceries, meeting childcare needs) without Marcus' support. Upon his release, as the realization set in that his return did not mean the end of the family's struggles, she became very disappointed. Marcus shared that he quickly became disappointed in himself, well-before Lisa expressed her feelings explicitly toward him. He shared that he currently feels like he doesn't know what to do, that he is in a lose-lose situation. The therapist encouraged Marcus to elaborate on what he meant by this. Marcus explained:

> The last thing I ever want is to become like my father and let my family down. I would rather drop dead than see them struggle and know it's my fault. But the thing is, that's what's already happening. I know I'm not actually going to die but I kinda feel like I'm dying on the inside. I could try and get back in the game, just for a little bit, just enough for us to get back on our feet and until we find a better solution, and then I know my family would be alright. But if I get caught, and go back to prison, then I'm definitely not going to be able to take care of my family. So I lose either way.

Through the sharing of his story, Lisa recognized how much Marcus was suffering as a result of not being able to fill the shoes he expected himself to, those which she as well expected him to fill. This metaphor came up one session and proved further helpful in deconstructing the way in which Lisa understood how her way of relating to Marcus affected him, in that, she soon came to the realization that although she may not have been the one who first brought these shoes before Marcus and asked him to wear them, she at no point asked him if they fit properly or if maybe they had become worn out and he needed a new pair.

Utilizing the same metaphor, Marcus recognized that these were shoes given to him as a child, and that it would be only natural for one to need to replace a pair of worn-out shoes they had been wearing now for decades. So used to the discomfort he experienced wearing these worn-out shoes however, Marcus was unable to recognize the need for a new pair, let alone communicate this to Lisa. And because Lisa could not know how uncomfortable these shoes were to Marcus, not wearing them herself, she had no way of knowing how much distress he was, and had no reason to consider that they may need to be replaced.

Through hearing Marcus relay his experiences growing up and how they impacted the way in which he viewed himself today and influenced the decisions he made, Lisa realized that she was not the protagonist of his story, but rather, he was. Although she was a main character, he was the only constant throughout the narrative he presented during session. She recognized that he was "subject" and she was "object". However, she had unknowingly, and without ill-intent, confused these designations, misperceiving herself to be the subject, and in the process, objectifying him. She realized that although their lives eventually overlapped at the time of their meeting, and therefore their stories did as well, they had not yet integrated the separate stories they brought with them to the relationship together, for the purpose of working out collaboratively a new story that they could share as a couple. A story that would see them both, together, as co-writers and co-protagonists.

In concurrence, Marcus realized that he was so narrowly focused on how badly he felt about himself and about how much he didn't want to let his family down, that he stopped paying attention to how they were *actually* doing and how they actually were affected by each one of his actions and decisions, rather than just how they *may* be affected in a general sense by his perceived shortcomings as a financial provider. He realized that instead of talking with Lisa, he just assumed he knew how she felt and what she was thinking. He explained how it now made sense to him that when she pulled away, he thought it was because she was getting ready to leave him, when it wasn't that at all. He had been in his own world so completely since he was released that he couldn't be present in theirs. Whereas Lisa downplayed Marcus' role of "subject" in his story, Marcus became too fixated on it, to the point that the other characters, his wife and his children, hardly existed. They too had their own stories in which they were protagonists, and he was just one of the main characters. He was so focused on his own story, however, that he went missing from theirs. Lisa too recognized that she was so preoccupied with her own experience, her own unmet expectations, that she failed to pay attention to how Marcus could have been struggling in his own way.

With a newly found understanding of and appreciation for one another's experiences and a recognition of their shared story of hardship, different in scope, but occurring within the context of the same events, the couple found a renewed sense of commitment to one another and a shared desire to overcome hardship. This experience was not unlike that of the first several years after they first met, but was even more akin to the first few years of Marcus' incarceration, when that commitment and shared sense of hopefulness carried them both through. Together, they would craft a third story in which both played equal parts in its writing, and both shared in the responsibility of working toward its realization.

At this point, the therapist pulled again from the Tadros Theory's incorporation of solution-focused techniques to help the couple maintain a forward-thinking perspective by assigning them homework to complete together. One assignment tasked them with making a list of "things that a family needs to be happy". The therapist stressed that this would require them to not be subjective and make a list of things that they as individuals *think* the other members of their family need, to not make a list based on assumptions, but to try and be as objective as possible, as broad and universal as possible. In the following session, the couple shared the list with the therapist and realized that, although some of the identified needs were dependent on maintaining a sufficient income, much of those needs, such as laughter, communication, connection, and love were going unmet as a result of Marcus and Lisa operating in isolation from one another, in pursuit of such things as fulfilling gender roles and attempting to meet unrealistic expectations for themselves and one another.

In between that session and the one planned for the following week, the therapist asked Marcus and Lisa to revisit the list and work together to figure out how they could each share the responsibility of making sure that these genuine needs were met and how they might go about doing it. When they returned, they shared that nearly all of the needs were found to be most realistically met if both shared in the responsibility, as partners, in doing so. Soon the couple developed the ability to problem solve collaboratively, to work together as a team to overcome the challenges their family faced, and to develop more realistic expectations for themselves and one another.

During future sessions, when the couple brought up issues that the family was facing, such as those related to financial difficulties, Marcus' difficulty in finding employment, or meeting childcare needs, they did so in ways that revealed an enormous decrease in the presence of blame in their relationship and a recognition of the reality of their situation, which allowed them to work as a team rather than as competitors, without keeping score of who was bringing what and how much to the relationship and to the family. This allowed the couple to focus on realistic and attainable solutions rather than to fixate on the problems they were facing. They had come to accept the barriers those with criminal records face when seeking employment as well as the impracticality of striving so rigidly toward meeting their shared expectation for Marcus to be the primary financial provider for the family.

The therapist made note of this development as it occurred over time and eventually brought these observations up to the couple, asking them to elaborate on how the couple experienced them in the home. Both Lisa and Marcus reported that they were experiencing an improved sense of well-being, mentally, emotionally, and relationally, and that they were much more satisfied with their relationship quality overall. They argued less, they laughed more, Marcus was more open and communicative, and Lisa was less critical. Based on their self-report, as well as on the therapist's observations about the couple's improved functioning as it presented during session, it was collaboratively determined that treatment had been a success and was subsequently terminated.

Case Example 2

Luke (35) and Michelle (34) are a Caucasian, working-class couple with a six-year-old daughter. Michelle works as a nurse and Luke formerly worked in an automotive manufacturing plant where he experienced a back injury during one of his shifts. Luke received worker's compensation but was unable to work for approximately six months while recovering and receiving treatment for his injury. As part of his treatment, Luke was prescribed opioid pain medication. Although he took the medication as prescribed, Luke eventually found it to be less and less effective over time. Periodically, the doctor would increase the dose to compensate for the natural tolerance Luke was developing.

Prior to returning to work, the doctor encouraged Luke to begin physical therapy to strengthen the muscles in his back, as a way to lessen his reliance on the injured portion which was causing him pain. The doctor then ceased the opioid medication and switched him to suboxone, as an opioid replacement therapy intended to slowly decrease his dependence on opiates while preventing withdrawal symptoms. Continued use of the opioid pain medication would have also prevented him from returning to work due to the dangers associated with operating heavy machinery while experiencing the medication's effects.

Luke quickly found that despite his pain being well managed and the suboxone being effective at eliminating his dependence on the pain medication, he missed its euphoric properties. Through mutual friends, he met someone who had access to opioid pain medications and sold them illicitly. Luke stopped the suboxone on his own, began abusing the pain medication he was obtaining off the street, while hiding this from Michelle and his doctor. Michelle had suspicions that something to this effect may have been occurring, but it wasn't until multiple accidents occurred at work due to Luke's negligence while under the influence that it became clear to Michelle and his employer that Luke was abusing opiates. Luke subsequently lost his job.

Michelle encouraged Luke to seek help, and he temporarily began the suboxone again. Luke struggled to remain clean. The only thing that did help him maintain stretches of time without using was the lack of income to purchase pain medications off the street. When able to afford it, he would stop the suboxone and return to using opiates. Eventually, Luke's persistent relapses led to full dependence on the opiates again. Luke began taking whatever measures necessary to obtain enough money to maintain this addiction, culminating in him attempting to rob a pharmacy of its opioid medications leading to his apprehension by the police in the process and subsequently being charged with second-degree robbery. Luke would spend four years in a state correctional facility.

Luke experienced a culture shock while in prison. He witnessed degrees of violence with which he had never been familiar and found it necessary to find a place within the hierarchy often found within incarceration facilities, involving fellow incarcerated individuals as well as correctional officers, if he wished to remain safe and to make his sentence as tolerable as possible. When Luke was eventually released, the impact this experience had on him could not be hidden. Luke was withdrawn, emotionally muted, unaffectionate, and reactive. Michelle was taken aback by what she recognized as a change in temperament and personality of the man that she had always loved. Michelle became fearful that Luke would begin using again if he had not done so already.

Soon after, Michelle became suspicious and intrusive. She frequently overwhelmed Luke, expressing concerns about his well-being and fears that he would relapse and again be re-incarcerated. Every time that Luke was scheduled to meet with his parole officer, she experienced, and expressed, anxieties that he would fail his routine drug tests, and she would lose him again. Although Michelle's concerns were valid and arose out of a genuine place of love and care, Luke did not feel supported and felt misunderstood. Luke did not want to begin using again; however, he felt like Michelle did not fully grasp the reality of his experience while incarcerated. Luke became further emotionally withdrawn and further closed off as a result. Luke opted to spend time with friends that he felt put less pressure on him, he was more comfortable being open with and, from his perspective, were less judgmental. As Luke drifted further away from Michelle, the greater her concerns grew about his potential drug use and the greater her inquisitions and intrusions became.

Luke eventually shared with his parole officer how much stress his relationship with Michelle was causing him and was in turn referred to couples therapy to address this turmoil. The therapist contacted Luke, approximately one week later, to schedule an initial session and to gather preliminary information about the difficulties he and Michelle had been facing. Luke was caught off guard by the phone call, having not once given thought to the prospect of participating in couples therapy since he spontaneously consented to his parole officer submitting a referral on his behalf just a week prior. Unsure of how to proceed and overwhelmed by the incursion of an unexpected phone call from a mental health provider, he quickly handed the phone over to Michelle, who already tended to hover over him whenever he was on the phone, out of anxiety over with whom he may be speaking and what about, simply saying to her, “some counselor is on the phone, you talk to them”, before immediately leaving the room.

Michelle shared with the therapist that Luke had recently been released from state prison after serving 4 years, explaining a bit about his charges, subsequent conviction, and the circumstances leading up to it. She shared that since Luke returned, he has been unusually quiet and “sneaky”. She shared that when he was initially incarcerated, he did seem somewhat sad and nervous on the phone and during in-person visits, but that he eventually began acting like the Luke she knew before the back injury and before his addiction began. She almost forgot that this was who he really is, she continued and was very excited for him to be released so they could resume the life they once shared together but had put on pause. She confessed that part of her was even glad he had gotten arrested at that point, that this could have been the opportunity needed for Luke to get his life back on track. However, when he returned home, things changed, she said. Luke wasn’t interested in talking much about anything really and rarely smiled or joked around with her like he used to, both before his addiction and during the latter half of his sentence. He helped with their daughter but never appeared excited to be around her or to initiate interactions with her, contrary to her assumption that he would want to make up for the lost years of witnessing her grow up.

Additionally, Luke was seldomly affectionate toward Michelle which devastated her, having gone without sex for four years while eagerly awaiting his release. She feared that maybe she had aged over those four years in such a way that he was no longer attracted to her. Ultimately, however, she expressed most concern over the possibility that Luke had begun abusing painkillers again, or if he had not yet, that he would soon. She shared that she worried almost constantly over this, but especially when Luke would leave, presumably to hang out with old friends; “but who really knows what he’s doing when he disappears like that?”, she then remarked. No matter how much she tried to talk to him, no matter how she went about doing it, she told the therapist, he never gave her much of anything at all that would provide insight into what was going on with him, what he was doing when he wasn’t home, and why he was acting so differently. Instead, he only ignored her or became irritable, eventually snapping at her succinctly, before removing himself from the situation, by either locking himself in their bedroom or leaving the house entirely. Michelle knew that if Luke began using again, he would without question be sent back to prison. She was terrified of this and did not know what to do. The therapist scheduled an initial session with the couple for the following week, requesting that Michelle confirm with Luke that he was willing to attend, and to reach back out if there were a need to reschedule.

For the initial session with the couple, the therapist sought to foster a safe environment in which sufficient space was provided for Luke to share his experience. The therapist was cognizant of how their previous phone conversation with Michelle could potentially hinder the development of a therapeutic alliance with Luke, given that a level of rapport had been established with Michelle already, whereas Luke entered the therapy room having not yet interacted with the therapist in any significant capacity. The therapist desired to offset this potential imbalance. Additionally, the therapist remained aware that although Michelle may have been speaking honestly and with sincerity during their conversation, there was certainly much about Luke's inner experience both during his incarceration and after his release that Michelle would have had no way of communicating to the therapist, thus providing the therapist with a biased and incomplete narrative of the problem as it presented itself in Luke and Michelle's relationship. The therapist desired to acquire a more well-rounded, more accurate understanding of the issues they were facing. In the process of becoming more familiar with the presenting problem, the therapist would be better able to make a decision on the most appropriate therapeutic intervention to utilize when treating the couple.

During the session, the therapist recapped the most pertinent points discussed during their conversation with Michelle to create an atmosphere of transparency, ensuring that Luke was made aware of the information that had already been disclosed. The therapist shared that they were aware of the events leading up to Luke's incarceration and that Michelle reported what she observed to be shifts in Luke's personality and demeanor, ultimately causing her concern that he may begin using opiates again. In summation, Michelle desired a stronger connection with Luke. The therapist inquired as to whether any of this was new information to Luke and if he had any thoughts about Michelle's disclosure. Luke shared that he was well aware of Michelle's opinions about him as she is reminding him of them daily. When offered opportunities to discuss the impact of Michelle's concerns on him and whether he felt as though her assessment of him was accurate, Luke chose not to elaborate or provide any strong thoughts or feelings one way or the other. Eventually, Michelle became visibly frustrated with Luke's apparent lack of engagement and began comparing his disposition during the session to "how he always is". As Michelle continued, Luke became visibly tense and appeared uncomfortable. The therapist acknowledged Michelle's frustration and pointed out Luke's discomfort which prompted him to finally express himself with exasperation, remarking that she "always gets like this" and that "it's exhausting". "It's too much to put up with", he concluded. The therapist thanked them for their willingness to share themselves in such a vulnerable way and their shared desire to come to therapy for the sake of one another and their relationship. A second session was scheduled for the following week.

Based on the information provided by both Luke and Michelle, as well as a pursuer-withdrawer dynamic that was present during the initial session–specifically when Luke refrained from engaging fully, prompting Michelle to react with frustration and Luke, in response, to express fatigue over her reaction–the therapist determined that utilizing Emotionally Focused Couple Therapy (EFT) as the modality of treatment would be most appropriate and most effective at treating the couple and their presenting problems (Johnson & Greenberg, 1985).

EFT was first formulated by Greenberg and Johnson in the 1980s and was grounded in attachment theory as well as developed from both experiential therapy and systemic structural therapy (Johnson, 2020). As are pertinent to the role a therapist plays when working with a couple, EFT inherited many of the tenets inherent in the experiential tradition, which focus on establishing a strong therapeutic alliance with all participants, the fostering of a safe environment to explore their emotional experiences within the therapy room, the acceptance and validation of these experiences as they are expressed by both partners, and the innate ability of both partners to become, not only aware of these experiences and expressions, but to also make conscious choices about whether they will continue expressing themselves as such or they will opt instead to behave and communicate in alternative ways (Johnson et al., 2022).

Given that the dynamics present in Luke and Michelle's relationship, as they emerged in session, mirrored the way they manifest themselves in the home, the therapist concluded that examining them and exploring the nature of them, along with the secondary as well as primary emotions that laid beneath them, in the safety of the therapeutic setting, would offer the couple an opportunity to evaluate and assess their usefulness in achieving the relational harmony the therapist suspected they both sought. In the process, the couple would be assisted in increasing their awareness of the negative patterns they found themselves trapped in and the role each played in the interactions that drove these patterns. Through the heightening of this awareness, and through the exploratory process of uncovering their negative interaction patterns, the therapist would engage the clients in such a way that would encourage them to consider a new mode of relating to and interacting with one another.

Furthermore, the therapist found EFT to be the most appropriate mode of intervention due to the influence that systemic techniques, most markedly those introduced by Minuchin in his structural therapeutic approach, have had on its development (Johnson et al., 2022). The therapist recognized early on that both Luke and Michelle were responding to each other in repeated negative loops where the more that Luke withdrew, the more that Michelle pursued him. And as Michelle's pursuit of Luke intensified, so did his withdrawal from and his avoidance of her. The structural technique of facilitating *enactments* during session would also help the couples stay in the present emotionally with each other and practice to communicate in a more accepting and bonding way. Therefore, the dynamic or interaction patterns could be shifted and the clients become engaged in practicing new patterns (Johnson, 2020).

Lastly, EFT's foundation of attachment theory would prove beneficial to the therapist in treating the couple, given that both were functioning within the context of a highly stressful period in their lives, adjusting to Luke's return to the home after having spent 4 years incarcerated. Bowlby (1969) introduced attachment theory in a humanistic and depathologizing manner, emphasizing that attachment behaviors are intrinsic to human beings, driving them to seek proximity with their attachment figures. According to Bowlby (1973), the presence of attachment figures diminishes fear-inducing conditions, while their absence amplifies them. In situations in which levels of stress are high, such as the one Luke and Michelle found themselves in, the greater there is a need for members of a relationship to feel secure in their bond with one another (Johnson et al., 2022). Yet, the disconnect between the couple, due to their separation and vastly different experiences during this period of separation, had eroded their bond, rendering them incapable of relying on one another for support and security as they navigated this transitional period in their lives. Feeling unable to rely on Michelle to cope with the difficult emotions he was experiencing post-release, Luke became avoidant in an act of self-preservation. In response, this avoidance triggered a heightened level of anxiety in Michelle, who in turn coped by pursuing Luke out of fear that their already insecure bond would further weaken.

The following few sessions the therapist placed great emphasis on building a strong therapeutic alliance with both Luke and Michelle independently until the strength of these respective alliances were sufficiently comparable that there were no longer two alliances held with each partner independently, but instead a single alliance held with them as a couple. This was an ongoing process occurring "in the background" while the therapist spent time learning about the couple's history from both Luke and Michelle's perspective. There were few points of contention between them until the point in their history after Luke was fired from his job and before he was arrested. This is the point at which Michelle reported Luke to have begun deliberately hiding things from her and lying about his drug use. The therapist asked Michelle if she knew at the time what was going on or if she only learned about it later. She shared that she knew at the time. She explained that it was different after he lost his job because before that she had just assumed he had been weaned off the pain medications and that was the end of it. Once he lost his job however, she reported being more vigilant and paid closer attention now that she knew he really was struggling with an actual addiction.

At this point in the session, the therapist began utilizing several techniques integral to EFT. They utilized evocative responding to encourage the couple to share their experiences on a deeper emotional level than they may have typically been inclined. The therapist employed extensive validation techniques to maintain the alliance and to foster a safe environment, ensuring that each client would feel comfortable continuing to express themselves in ways that they might otherwise avoid out of fear of judgment or rejection. The therapist also offered up alternative ways of understanding their own and each other's emotional experiences, proposing that certain more vulnerable emotions may have actually been present but masked by less self-threatening, secondary emotions such as anger. While doing so, the therapist utilized the technique of heightening through repetitive use of words, phrases, emotions, and themes to bring both Luke and Michelle deeper into their lived experience (Johnson et al., 2022).

The therapist asked Luke if he could tell that Michelle was keeping a closer eye on him after he lost his job and what that was like. Luke shared that he felt like he was under constant surveillance from her and it "irritated the hell out of [him]". The therapist asked him how he would react when he felt irritated and Luke shared that at first, he tried to play it off by lying to her, or by making excuses to explain his behaviors. Eventually, however, Luke reported growing impatient with her over time, to the point that he would scream and curse at her to try and get her to just leave him alone. The therapist validated these emotions and normalized his reactions without condoning the behavior, doing so by acknowledging the insidiousness of addiction, acknowledging that it often takes over a person's life and anything that might interfere with maintaining the addiction could be seen as a threat. Therefore, it all adds up that he might try and hide things from her or lie to her, even react with hostility. The therapist then pivoted to Michelle and asked her what it was like for her to see this going on right in front of her eyes but without having any way to prove it. They inquired what it was like to have Luke constantly deny what was going on every time she confronted him about it, even though she knew he was lying, and then what it was like for her when he would become angry.

Michelle shared that at first, she felt reassured when he would lie to her or offer an explanation for suspicious behaviors as she didn't want to believe that he was still abusing drugs. However, when she could no longer pretend that this wasn't the case, she became angry herself. Angry, she said, because it was if he thought she was stupid enough to believe him and because she just wanted him to admit to her what he was doing. She just wanted him to be honest and it "pissed her off" that he never was, even though it was so obvious to her what he was doing.

The therapist asked her to consider whether she might have been fearful in the beginning, fearful of what it would mean if Luke had begun using again, and if it were possible that his lies made her fearfulness go away. The therapist continued offering considerations by asking if she may have felt disrespected or even betrayed that Luke refused to be truthful with her even though it was so obvious to her what was going on. She acknowledged that she was very afraid at the time and that she still is but was mostly confused with who this person she thought she knew and loved had become and that that just made her incredibly angry. "So, the person you fell in love with turned out not to be who you thought he was?", the therapist inquired. Michelle explained that she knows he's the same person and that the drugs were just making him act differently, but at the time she wasn't sure. "So, you felt misled in a way? Deceived? Possibly betrayed even?", the therapist asked. Michelle embraced this perspective in agreement.

The therapist then asked Luke what else may have been going on with him, besides irritation, when Michelle was constantly asking him questions and confronting him with suspicions about ongoing drug use. Luke shared that it felt like she didn't understand what he was going through, that he already felt like he was alone and couldn't trust anyone. He had recently just lost his job, he reminded the therapist, and everyone at work knew why. But now, even Michelle didn't understand him and, even though he now understands that this wasn't the case, at the time he just felt like she was constantly attacking him, criticizing him, treating him like he was "some kind of terrible person". He was embarrassed, he shared, when he lost his job, and he felt ashamed that he kept using drugs anyway. Luke then shared that even though he doesn't feel as though Michelle is as critical of him or is as attacking as she was back then, he still feels like she treats him as if he is still using drugs, that he still can't be trusted, and like he is still under, what feels like to him, constant surveillance.

"It can be very, very lonely when nobody understands what we're going through", the therapist acknowledged. "It can also be incredibly scary", they continued, "to feel like we're under constant threat of criticism and to have to face our problems alone. It can also be terrifying to care about someone so much and to see them struggling. Especially when we don't know how to help them".

The therapist ended the session by proposing that both Luke and Michelle were both very afraid for very different but both very valid reasons at this period in their lives. They also both experienced feeling cut off from one another, believing that either the other was out to get them, didn't understand them, or that their partner was not who they had always believed them to be. Both Luke and Michelle, the therapist shared with the couple, must have felt very alone and very confused. And both those emotions can make a person very fearful. "When we're afraid", the therapist concluded, "we often behave in ways that don't always make sense to ourselves or to the people around us, until we look back on it after some time has passed and have a different vantage point from which to understand it".

Having spent the initial few sessions learning about the couple's history and familiarizing themselves with the context within which their current problems arose, the therapist sought next to explore what their interactions looked like in the present and the emotions they typically expressed to one another as these interactions were occurring, doing so through the continued use of the EFT techniques they had utilized so far. Luke had previously mentioned feeling in some ways like Michelle still treats him the way she did before his arrest, when he was actively using. The therapist reminded the couple of Luke's comparison and gave Michelle an opportunity to also describe their current interactions as they do or do not share similarities with that period of time.

Michelle shared that she was currently similarly concerned for Luke's well-being, as she had been after he lost his job, and although she didn't necessarily believe that Luke was actively using again, the thought that he may be never left her mind. Instead, she more so feared that, if he weren't using already, that could change on any given day, and aside from the impact that that would have on his health and well-being, as well as the impact it would have on their relationship, it could also lead to his re-incarceration.

"Aside from the obvious, that you care for him, and he of course has abused substances in the past, what is it today that leads you to believe that he *could* be using again? What is it that causes you to be so concerned that, if he isn't already, it's only a matter of time before he is?", the therapist asked Michelle.

"Well, I knew he wasn't using when he was in jail", she explained, "because how was he going to get anything? And it's not like he had much money even if he could find drugs. I had a really hard time affording the phone calls already, on top of our usual bills and everything else, so it's not like I was able to put a ton of money on his commissary account too. But really it was just the way he acted when me and our daughter would visit. Sure, in the beginning he seemed off, he was still getting used to being there, but eventually he seemed almost happy even. He would smile the whole time we were together; he would make jokes, he asked me how things were at home, and tell me how much he was looking forward to getting out and basically just starting a new chapter in our lives. I don't know, I could just tell".

"And now you can't", the therapist responded. "What's different?" "Everything", Michelle immediately replied, before continuing:

> He never asks me how I am or how my day was. He never laughs or tries to make me laugh, and when he does smile, which is almost never, you can tell he's forcing it just to be polite or to try and make it seem like everything is fine. Like if I ask him what's wrong and he tells me that nothing's wrong, he sometimes fakes a smile as if he's trying to cover something up or convince me that everything really is fine. That almost never happens anymore though. Now if I try and talk to him, ask him what's bothering him or what he's doing, where he's going when he leaves the house, or if there's something I should be worried about, he usually just ignores me or snaps at me. If I don't just leave him alone at that point, he'll go lock himself in our room or just leave the house altogether.

"And this is what it was like after he lost his job, when he was using, right before he got arrested?", the therapist inquired. Michelle replied:

> Well, back then, eventually he didn't even try to hide it. And it didn't matter what I said or did, he would come and go as he pleased and act like me and our daughter didn't even exist. If I did say something to him about it though, he would get really angry and yell over me until I gave up, or he left. But before it got to that point, even before he lost his job and it became obvious that he was still using, yeah, it's just like that. He seemed far away, like he does now. There was no arguing as long as he was left alone, but he never seemed interested in me or our daughter or really anything at all. He doesn't give me much if anything just like before. If I ask him something, it's like he's trying to answer me in as few of words as possible. And so yeah, it makes me think he's using again. The only thing that convinces me that he's not is he keeps passing his drug tests. But I'm just waiting for the day that he doesn't.

"I can see why you would be so concerned, so fearful. It sounds like you're very afraid.", the therapist responded. "Luke", they continued, "what's all this like for you? You must know Michelle is worried about you, is that how it comes across? Do you think she has a reason to be worried?"

"I don't know, honestly", Luke began, before pausing for a few moments and then continuing:

> It's like, sure yeah, she doesn't want me to start using again, and I get that, and I really screwed things up big time for our family, I mean, there's a reason I was in prison for 4 years. But I'm not using, and I'm not going to, and I don't know how many times I have to tell her that before she'll

> believe me. I really don't know what I'm supposed to do. I've been trying to get a job, which is difficult with a record. I've been helping with our daughter. I've been doing everything my parole officer tells me to do, and I pass all my drug tests. She's constantly questioning me, non-stop though, it never ends and it's like I have no space ever and it gets to be so annoying that yeah, eventually I do lose my temper and tell her to "shut-up" or "leave me alone" and I know I shouldn't and I don't like doing it so instead I just leave the house now and go for a drive or hang out with one of my friends, or even just go into our bedroom and, yeah, lock the door so she can't bother me. She might be worried about me, but the way she's going about it isn't doing anything but stressing me out.

"But you were like this as soon as you came home", Michelle interjected, "before I even started to ask you if you were getting high again".

"It still felt like you were always hovering over me though, right from the beginning, it was like everything I said or did, you would like, analyze my facial expressions, always asking me what was wrong or if everything was okay. It felt like you were trying to read my thoughts. It was too much. Sometimes I just need space". Luke responded.

"It sounds to me like Luke's release has required a lot of adjusting, for both of you", the therapist remarked. They continued:

> Four years is a long time to be away from someone, just to suddenly one day be reunited. I'm sure both of you were looking forward to it and maybe even were very hopeful. Luke, you finally got to go home and experience freedom again, the comfort of your own space and your own bed. You could finally be with Michelle, your daughter, and see your friends again. And Michelle, you got Luke back, a clean and sober Luke, the person he was before the accident, before the drugs, before your lives were turned upside down. You no longer had to do it all alone anymore. But even though you both might have hoped things could go back to the way they were before all of that, you two went through a lot while you were separated and lived two very different lives while you were apart. Maybe you two need to "get to know each other" again.

"I'm so happy to have Luke back", Michelle said. "You have no idea how difficult it was while he was away and how much I missed him. It's just, it's like, even though he's here now, it's like he never came back".

"Luke, what about you?", the therapist asked.

"I'm sure it was difficult for her trying to get by all on her own. But also, I was in prison. Do you know what that's like? She has no idea what that was like. But it's my fault I ended up there, I know that, so I don't bring it up. I don't need anyone feeling sorry for me".

Luke eventually shared that he witnessed many things in prison which he found disturbing and that he had to become a different person, in a way, just to blend in and, as he described it, "survive". In preparation for the next session, the therapist constructed a visual depiction of the negative interaction cycle, an integral component of EFT, to share with the couple and to help them become aware of the dynamics of their relationship, for the purpose of empowering them to better understand one another and to make the necessary changes to improve the quality of it (Johnson, 2020).

The next session, the therapist presented the negative interaction cycle to the couple and explained to them what it represented and the significance of it. They explained that both Luke and Michelle harbored deep feelings of fear for reasons specific to them. Michelle was fearful that Luke was hiding things from her, that he would begin using again, and that he would be re-incarcerated and she would once again lose him. She also felt sadness and loneliness that their connection was not what it once was, nor what she imagined it would be when he was released. Luke was fearful of what his experience in prison meant for how he viewed himself and fearful that Michelle might view him differently as well. Luke as well experienced feelings of sadness and loneliness manifesting out of his discomfort with engaging in emotional intimacy with Michelle.

The therapist helped the couple recognize how their attachment orientations impact, and play out cyclically through, their interactions with one another. The therapist validated these emotions, acknowledging that they can be very difficult for a person to experience, and that one can feel threatened, at risk of harm, if these emotions persist. Therefore, to protect ourselves, we often allow "safer", "stronger" emotions to take over which we then express and act on. These emotions mask our true experience and can give way to conflict with others. In the case of Michelle, the therapist explained that she experienced suspicion (of what Luke was doing), and anger, for him not communicating more openly with her. Anger for making her feel afraid, even. She also experienced anxiety, constant worrying and fixating over "what if's". This led her to seek constant reassurance from Luke that he was not using, it caused her to mistrust what he did and said, and it prompted her to become invasive and pursue him endlessly, both with questions and through close physical proximity.

Luke's underlying feelings of fear, loneliness, and sadness, were masked by feelings of shame for what he had seen and what he had done while incarcerated, by frustration and irritability with Michelle, for making it so difficult for him to withhold that which he preferred not to look at nor show to her, as well as by anxiety, which he experienced when Michelle was too persistent in her pursuits. In coping with these emotions, Luke withdrew himself from Michelle, choosing to isolate out of fear that he would be rejected or misunderstood. He significantly limited his communication with her and avoided her when he felt that what she was asking of him was something he was unable to give her due to the anxiety it caused him. Finally, he would become reactive, expressing his frustration and irritability with her when his efforts to avoid her failed.

Bowlby (1973) indicated that accessibility as well as responsiveness shaped how people view themselves and the world they are in. In light of this, the therapist shared that both Luke and Michelle ultimately wanted the same thing from one another, connection and acceptance. It is natural for people to expect their attachment figures to be generally responsive and available to support them occasionally or most of the time, which shapes both their sense of self-worthiness as well as security (Bowlby, 1973). Missing from their relationship, however, was an adequate level of trust necessary for this connection to occur. Michelle wanted to trust that Luke wasn't going to be taken away from her again and that he still was in love with her. Luke wanted to trust that Michelle wouldn't judge him, that she would be patient with him as he adjusted after his release, and that she would accept him as he was. However, due to this lack of trust, Luke withdrew from Michelle to avoid the possibility that these things he desired would not be given to him. In turn, due to her lack of trust in him, Michelle pursued Luke in an effort to obtain the level of connection she desired and to placate the lack of trust present. However, the more Michelle pursued Luke out of fear, the more he pulled away out of his own fear. And as Luke's efforts to withdraw himself from Michelle persisted, Michelle's pursuit of him proved only to grow greater. As a result, neither were getting what they wanted out of their relationship, and in fact, were getting just the opposite.

The therapist offered them the perspective that this cycle was something they were unknowingly and unintentionally perpetuating in unison while, as a result, both suffering from it together. Luke and Michelle were not at odds with one another, instead, they were together at odds with the cycle. The goal, which the therapist offered to help them achieve, was to interrupt this cycle and address the underlying emotions that the cycle had so effectively hidden beneath it, so that both could learn to trust one another enough to establish the connection with and sense of security in one another they both sought.

Having identified and subsequently shared with Luke and Michelle the negative interaction cycle present in their relationship, and in the process assisting them in recognizing the underlying emotions and unmet needs which, being unresolved, give way to the behaviors that perpetuate the cycle, the therapist proceeded to assist the couple as they got in touch with these emotions and needs in a more lived-in way, so that they could be communicated with one another, and the cycle interrupted. In the following sessions, the therapist continued to utilize interventions integral to EFT.

The therapist later focused on enactment to shape the new interaction patterns, and heightened the experiences of fear and loneliness that had been revealed to exist within both Luke and Michelle, but previously hidden from both themselves and from one another. The therapist did this by encouraging each to share with one another in session when and how these emotions arose and how it influenced the way they had been interacting with one another since Luke's release.

"It sounds like when Michelle asks you how you're doing or if everything is okay", the therapist spoke to Luke, "you experience discomfort because you are fearful that if you answer her truthfully, she wouldn't understand and might not accept you. That sounds terrifying. Could you turn to Michelle and tell her that you want to be open and honest with her, but you're afraid that if you are, you might lose her?" The therapist then reframed the behaviors that followed these emotions to adjust the way Michelle understands Luke's avoidance of her and soften any negative emotions she may feel in response.

"You run away from Michelle not because you don't love her, not because you are afraid of connection, no. You run away from Michelle because you're afraid if she really saw you up close, she wouldn't love you anymore. You run away not because you're afraid of connection, but because you are afraid of losing what little connection you have left".

The therapist utilized these same interventions while engaging with Michelle, saying to her, "When you feel Luke pull away, when you feel shut out by him, it horrifies you. You're horrified because it reminds you of how you felt when he was using, and you know what happened next. You want to trust him, but you need him to reassure you that this is not what is happening. When he says nothing, you can only go off what you've known before, what past experience dictates. Can you tell him that you want to trust him, but it's so difficult for you, because you're so afraid of losing him again?"

The therapist continued this chain of interventions by reframing Michelle's anger, speaking to her, "When you become suspicious of Luke, sometimes frustrated, even accusatory, you're not actually angry with him, you're angry with your unresolved feelings of fear. You feel as though Luke could take those feelings of fear away from you if only, if only he opened up to you and shared with you what is going on with him. You think, 'this could all be so easy, all you have to do is talk to me and I won't be afraid anymore!', but when this doesn't happen you become angry. Angry at this fear that won't leave you. And because that fear still lingers, you attempt to resolve it in other ways, by pursuing Luke, by questioning him, by constantly 'looking over his shoulder', if you will".

"Luke", the therapist asked, "what is it like for you when you withdraw from Michelle to avoid losing her, but she follows right behind you?"

"Well, I get anxious and honestly, I get mad and snap at her because all I want is my space and she isn't giving it to me", Luke said.

The therapist responded, "It sounds like, just like Michelle pursues you as a way to cope with her fear, you withdraw from her to cope with yours.

And just as she pursues you out of fear that she may lose you, you pull away from her out of fear that you could lose her as well. Could you turn to Michelle and tell her that you're afraid of losing her?"

Next, the therapist worked with the couple to identify new ways of responding to their difficult emotions and in the process helped them restructure and reshape their interactions, to better address their feelings of fear and mistrust, as well as their needs related to attachment. The therapist began this by asking Luke what he needs from Michelle when he feels that fear that makes him withdraw from her. He shared that he needs space and patience. The therapist then asked Michelle what she would need from Luke to respect those wishes. Reassurance, she said. Reassurance that he would eventually come back to her to share with her what he was feeling and why, as well as reassurance that he wasn't going to be using drugs while he was away.

When Michelle shared this, the therapist noticed Luke tense up a bit and therefore utilized the EFT interventions of tracking, reflecting, and replaying.

"Luke", the therapist stepped in, "when Michelle shared something she would like from you, that she would like you to eventually share your feelings and your thoughts with her, you seemed uneasy. Was that the fear popping back up again? The fear that if you do this she won't understand or accept you? The fear that you will lose her?"

Luke confirmed the accuracy of the therapist's observation.

The therapist continued, "Luke, could you remind Michelle that opening up to her is scary, but you want to do it anyway. Could you tell her that you need her help to overcome that fear? That you need her to reassure you that she loves you, that she won't judge you, and that you can trust her? That if you are going to open up to her, you need her simply to listen with compassion and understanding?"

After Luke had done this, the therapist turned to Michelle, asking, "Could you turn to Luke and offer him that reassurance now, Michelle?"

Continuing this process over the course of several sessions, the therapist was able to successfully achieve a major objective of EFT. Luke, who had previously withdrawn from the relationship, found himself in a position to define new terms by which Michelle would engage with him so that he would feel less fearful and more trusting of her. In exchange, Luke would take steps to interact with Michelle in a new way, a way in which he would help her alleviate her own feelings of fear and mistrust (Johnson, 2020).

Now that Luke and Michelle possessed a more empathetic understanding of one another's emotional experiences and were cognizant of each other's needs in the relationship, the therapist guided them as they collaboratively worked out a plan for how they would go about meeting those needs in a practical, concrete way. Michelle agreed to pay close attention to her anxiety level and recognize when she felt the urge to demand things from Luke, such as excessive reassurance or detailed information about his experience in an interrogative way. She would acknowledge and name her experience as being driven by fear and mistrust. In place of her old ways of coping, she would simply share with Luke that she was feeling afraid and that she would like him to help her overcome her fears.

In return, Luke agreed that he would not become defensive or immediately pull away. Instead, he would reassure her that her feelings were valid and that he was there to help her work through them. He would let her know whether he felt safe to talk with her at that moment or if not, what he needed to feel safe and when he felt like he would feel equipped to talk with her. They would remind one another of their shared desire for emotional connection and shared desire for mutual trust. Together they determined, if Luke was not prepared in the moment to engage in communication with Michelle, what a reasonable amount of time—given the circumstances, the intensity of one another's distress, and one another's schedules and plans for the day—would be to permit Luke to prepare himself, before agreeing to sit down with Michelle and work through the situation together.

Luke also agreed to work on maintaining the degree of self-awareness necessary to, when thoughts or feelings related to his incarceration came up, take note of them and reflect on their impact on him. He would remind himself that, holding these things in and erecting a barrier to keep Michelle out, would prevent him from obtaining the security and sense of safety in his connection with her that he desired. In those moments, he would let Michelle know, if she were present, simply that he was having difficult thoughts and feelings. He did not need to talk about them with her in the moment, but simply make her aware of this, so that she did not have to read into anything he said or did with a lack of information, which had traditionally led her to make assumptions that were almost always fear based, fears related to drug use and ultimately losing Luke. Luke would then spend some time considering what about those thoughts and feelings he felt comfortable sharing with Michelle and to what extent he was willing to elaborate on them. When he felt ready, he would remind Michelle that he needed her to listen and offer reassurance that he could trust her, that she would not judge his experience, nor press him to elaborate further than he felt comfortable, before then sharing with her those thoughts and feelings.

The therapist continued to meet with the couple for an additional four sessions to monitor and consolidate the change between them. The therapist congratulated them on their successes as they modified their interactions with one another, as well as encouraged them when they experienced challenges while assisting them in overcoming them. The therapist requested feedback from the couple regarding how they felt things were going at home in between sessions, whether they felt confident in themselves to navigate new situations as they arose, and whether the idea of ending therapy caused them any concern.

Rather soon after the therapist began tracking their feedback, Luke and Michelle shared that they were seeing positive changes in their relationship and felt prepared to continue the process that had begun in therapy independently, without the therapist's oversight or assistance. The therapist reminded the couple of how much has changed over the course of therapy and how far they had come since they initially began. They encouraged Luke and Michelle to keep implementing the new habits they have developed and reminded them that, although they would likely encounter bumps along the way, they possessed the skills necessary to overcome them together, while nonetheless offering to them the option to return at any point in the future for booster sessions, should they find themselves so derailed and in the midst of crises so great, that they believed themselves unable to navigate their way out on their own. With these parting words, treatment was officially terminated.

Potential Future Clinical and Research Avenues

Due to the limited research conducted on the impact of MFTs on improving relationship quality among couples affected by incarceration, both during the incarceration period and post-release, impacted as well by the absence of a well-established precedence of MFT involvement in treating couples comprising this population in general, proposals for such involvement must be informed by what relevant resources are available and what can be extrapolated from these resources.

The summaries of recommendations made by topical scholars as well as the two case illustrations previously provided satisfy this necessity and achieve this objective. It is the authors' conclusion that this information be put into practice and efforts be made to incorporate MFT involvement during the re-entry and post-release period for the purpose of assisting romantic partners affected by incarceration in reducing relationship conflict as well as the rate of relationship dissolution.

This chapter explored formerly incarcerated men who struggle to process and address feelings of inadequacy and shame related to their inability to serve as primary providers for their families, the guilt they experience as a result of their financial dependence on romantic partners both during and after incarceration, as well as the influence these uncomfortable emotions have on their subsequent actions. Men frequently cope with the guilt and shame by withdrawing from their partners and other family members, risking the sustainability of their relationship, and often will as well consider, if not follow through on, returning to criminal activities to generate income, running the risk of re-incarceration.

Conclusion

There is a rich and extensive catalog of research-informed literature on the impact of incarceration on the non-incarcerated family members, a substantial amount of which examines the negative impact on the romantic partners of the incarcerated individual. An apparent and irrefutable need for interventions to alleviate this impact is revealed as a result, leading scholars, policymakers, and researchers to bring attention to this need and recommend that it be addressed in broad fashion. Despite the presence of a diverse assortment of services, policy changes, and interventions having been proposed, none have considered creating opportunities MFTs to play a role in meeting this need. With the addition of this chapter to a pre-existing body of literature devoted to addressing the needs of this population, it is hoped that awareness of the positive impact MFT involvement would have will be raised, and the indisputability of this impact recognized.

References

Bowlby, J. (1969). *Attachment and loss, Vol. 1: Attachment. Attachment and loss.* Basic Books.

Bowlby, J. (1973). *Attachment and loss: Vol. 2. Separation, anxiety and anger.* Basic Books.

Cafferky, B. M., Mendez, M., Anderson, J. R., & Stith, S. M. (2018). Substance use and intimate partner violence: A meta-analytic review. *Psychology of Violence, 8*(1), 110–131. https://doi.org/10.1037/vio0000074

Charles, P., Muentner, L. D., & Kjellstrand, J. (2019). Parenting and incarceration: Perspectives on father-child involvement during reentry from prison. *Social Service Review, 93*(2), 218–261. https://doi.org/10.1086/703446

Comfort, M., Krieger, K. E., Landwehr, J., McKay, T., Lindquist, C. H., Feinberg, R., Kennedy, E. K., & Bir, A. (2018). Partnership after prison: Couple relationships during reentry. *Journal of Offender Rehabilitation, 57*(2), 188–205. https://doi.org/10.1080/10509674.2018.1441208

DeHart, D., Shapiro, C., & Clone, S. (2018). "The pill line is longer than the Chow Line": The impact of incarceration on prisoners and their families. *The Prison Journal, 98*(2), 188–212. https://doi.org/10.1177/0032885517753159

Hairston, C. F., & Oliver, W. (2006). Women's experiences with men's incarceration and reentry. *Women, Girls, & Criminal Justice, 7*(5), 65–80.

Harman, J. J., Smith, V. E., & Egan, L. C. (2007). The impact of incarceration on intimate relationships. *Criminal Justice and Behavior, 34*(6), 794–815. https://doi.org/10.1177/0093854807299543

Jalali, F., Hashemi, S., Kimiaei, S., Hasani, A., & Jalali, M. (2017). The effectiveness of solution -focused brief couple therapy on marital satisfaction among married prisoners and their wives. *International Journal of Offender Therapy and Comparative Criminology, 62*(10), 3023–3037. https://doi.org/10.1177/0306624x17733662

Johnson, S. M. (2020). *The practice of emotionally focused couple therapy: Creating connection* (Third ed.). Routledge. https://doi.org/10.4324/9781351168366

Johnson, S. M., & Greenberg, L. S. (1985). Emotionally focused couples therapy: An outcome study. *Journal of Marital and Family Therapy, 11*(3), 313–317. https://doi.org/10.1111/j.1752-0606.1985.

Johnson, S. M., Wiebe, S. A., & Allan, R. (2022). Emotionally focused couple therapy. In J. L. Lebow & D. K. Snyder (Eds.), *Clinical handbook of couple therapy* (6th ed., pp. 127–150). Guilford Publications.

McKay, T., Landwehr, J., Lindquist, C., Feinberg, R., Comfort, M., Cohen, J., & Bir, A. (2018). Intimate partner violence in couples navigating incarceration and reentry. *Journal of Offender Rehabilitation, 57*(5), 273–293. https://doi.org/10.1080/10509674.2018.1487897

Minuchin, S. (1974). *Families and family therapy.* Harvard College.

Negash, S., Chung, K., & Oh, S. (2022). Families post-release: Barriers and pathways to family therapy. *Family Process, 61*(2), 609–624. https://doi.org/10.1111/famp.12769

Stansfield, R., Mowen, T. J., Napolitano, L., & Boman, J. H. (2020). Examining change in family conflict and family violence after release from prison. *Criminal Justice and Behavior, 47*(6), 668–687. https://doi.org/10.1177/0093854820913311

Tadros, E. (2019). The Tadros Theory of change: An integrated structural, narrative, and solution-focused approach. *Contemporary Family Therapy, 41*(4), 347–356. https://doi.org/10.1007/s10591-019-09502-z

Tadros, E. (2021). The Tadros Theory of change with incarcerated populations. *The American Journal of Family Therapy, 50*(4), 368–388. https://doi.org/10.1080/01926187.2021.1929560

Tadros, E., & Smithee, L. C. (2022). Treating incarcerated lesbian couples with the Tadros Theory of Change. *Journal of Gay & Lesbian Social Services, 34*(1), 63–85. https://doi.org/10.1080/10538720.2021.1921649

Turney, K. (2015). Hopelessly devoted? Relationship quality during and after incarceration. *Journal of Marriage and Family, 77*(2), 480–495. https://doi.org/10.1111/jomf.12174

Zamble, E., & Porporino, F. (1990). Coping, imprisonment, and rehabilitation. *Criminal Justice and Behavior, 17*(1), 53–70. https://doi.org/10.1177/0093854890017001005

Chapter 10

Family Reunification

Coparents Post-Release

Jeffrey Shewell and Eman Tadros

As made evident in the previous chapter, which explored the experiences of romantic couples during the period after which one member of the partnership was released from a correctional facility, unique challenges arise within relationships affected by incarceration. The chapter also demonstrated how marriage and family therapists (MFTs) can play a pivotal role in helping these couples overcome such challenges. One aspect of these relationships, however, that the previous chapter did not explore is how dyads, whether still romantically involved or not, navigate issues surrounding coparenting, when the pair shares one or more children together. This chapter will explore this important topic and how MFTs can be utilized to facilitate these negotiations using relational therapy. Relational therapy aims to assist people who are having difficulty developing and maintaining stable, healthy, and safe relationships.

Most people who have or currently are, coparenting, are keenly aware of differences on how to approach the variety of issues or situations that sometimes arise between caregivers while parenting. After all, what child has not at some point deliberately asked one parent over the other for something, knowing from past experience that this parent would be the one more likely to say yes? Or what of the child who has gotten into trouble and is particularly more afraid to face one parent over the other, because they are historically more strict and less likely to grant concessions than their counterpart? And for those among us who are parents, who have not at times disagreed with their partner over such seemingly consequential but oftentimes ultimately trivial matters as determining the ideal bedtime, granting appropriate privileges related to spending time with friends, or establishing appropriate consequences for misbehavior? Sometimes though, the disagreements are intentionally avoided altogether by one partner deferring to and relinquishing all decision-making power to the other caregiver! In these instances, despite the presence of two parents, one could hardly call this arrangement coparenting. The potential for disagreements over parenting

DOI: 10.4324/9781003542940-10

however is ever present, although certainly more so pronounced in some families than in others.

Different stances that parents take in the raising of their children can be easily resolved at times, while at others, they become inflated, ballooning until conflict erupts. In the case of parents where one was recently released from a correctional facility, there exist even more opportunities for a difference in stances to escalate into serious disagreements or conflict. Because, although the need to develop an appropriate bedtime or determine appropriate privileges for a child of a particular age are still relevant in these cases, it is not unusual for the non-incarcerated caregiver to believe that the recently released parent shouldn't even have a say in these matters to begin with, dependent of course on how long they were absent due to incarceration. In such cases, a disagreement about bedtime turns into a disagreement about who has the authority to even make the decision. It becomes a disagreement about a disagreement!

This chapter will shed light on common issues related to the topic of coparenting, which present when one caregiver reenters society after a period of incarceration. Data shows this parent tends to be male, so we will be using the masculine, but we acknowledge that an increasing number of mothers have been incarcerated (Ghandnoosh et al., 2021). Broadly speaking, many of these issues are rooted in disagreements between caregivers over how and to whom the roles and responsibilities necessitated by coparenting children are delegated. More specifically, these disagreements occur when considering such things as who is responsible for childcare and supervision or who possesses the authority to make decisions about how a child is reared. But additionally, questions related to the trustworthiness of the recently released parent and feelings of ambivalence about their ability to ensure the safety of a child, sometimes present within this population, will be posed as well.

Given that a strong case has already been made for the efficacy, and therefore necessity, of the involvement of MFTs during the reentry period to improve the outcomes of romantic relationships, the benefits inherent in their involvement for the purpose of establishing an effective coparenting relationship between caregivers can be easily recognized. A reliance on evidence presented in the previous chapter will be built off of with new information introduced to further substantiate the claim that MFTs could play a pivotal role in nurturing and strengthening coparenting relationships post-incarceration in individual, couple, and family therapy. This chapter will discuss what should be focused on in treatment post-release and how to make the bridge from therapy inside to therapy outside.

Finally, a case study will be presented which depicts coparents as they struggle to amicably and collaboratively navigate common issues faced by this population, with an example of what an intervention performed by

MFTs might look like, further demonstrating the critical need for their involvement, and supporting the call for the widespread use of therapeutic interventions in the interest of overcoming challenges faced by coparents during the post-release period.

Changing of the Guard

The previous chapter briefly examined the impact that an individual's incarceration may have on their partner's financial stability, as well as the difficulties that arise when two available caregivers become only one. A consequence of incarceration can be a non-incarcerated partner suddenly beginning to function like a single parent in various aspects, singularly responsible for ensuring childcare is available in order to avoid almost certain unemployment; an inevitability emerging out of the need to guarantee that any child requiring it is provided with adequate supervision at all times.

The chapter then explored the emotional fallout that follows these consequences, the guilt and shame the incarcerated partner often feels and the anger and resentment the female partner develops in kind. The hope she holds onto, the hope that her partner's release will alleviate the financial burdens caused by his incarceration, however, frequently goes unfulfilled, almost exclusively due to the barriers to employment he now faces with a criminal record and his financial dependence on her.

However, despite what would appear here to be a naturally occurring, reasonably assumed, and mutually agreed upon arrangement, the reality instead is that the incarcerated partner's release does not always relieve the existing challenges associated with the need for childcare. In fact, it sometimes is the case that, rather than offering a solution to the problem of childcare, reentry instead merely transforms the nature of the problem into one equally challenging and in just as much need of overcoming as it did in its previous form, as it existed pre-release. No longer is the problem a matter of lacking options for childcare; now it's a matter of *whose* responsibility it is to provide childcare. Barriers to easily settling this debate take the form of assumptions held, expectations challenged, senses of entitlement, and the corresponding conflict, which ultimately can and does arise as a result.

Comfort et al. (2018) highlight the case of one man recently released from an incarceration facility who soon found himself stuck at home all day caring for his children while his partner worked, something that would have previously been difficult for her without the childcare assistance the man could now provide. The man likened the experience to being locked up again, wishing instead to begin reestablishing a life for himself, something he could not do until he was released. Given that many women must put their lives on hold, set their careers aside, become financially independent, and struggle to maintain steady employment functioning as single parents, the release of the incarcerated parent opens up new opportunities for them, allowing them to take advantage of their partner's availability to provide childcare, having eagerly anticipated their release for this very purpose. The recently released partners, however, feel similarly, in that their newly obtained freedom offers them an opportunity as well to reestablish a life, to reenter the workforce, and reconnect with friends and family. Disagreements between the caregivers over who is now more entitled to take advantage of these newly offered opportunities may emerge.

Consequently, the question arises: Who has given up more, and therefore, who is now more entitled to benefit from the newfound sense of freedom and opportunity that the post-release period provides? The previously incarcerated partner (most often discussed as a cis-gender man) was deprived of his liberty in many aspects of existence while confined behind the walls of a correctional facility. And, although he may have missed his children profoundly and may possess great feelings of guilt over his absence in their lives, upon his release, is it not unreasonable for him to desire a period of time in which he is not responsible for the welfare of others, but instead afforded the opportunity to explore the liberties, previously deprived of him, now available to him post-incarceration?

Comparably, the female caregiver also served a sentence, different in nature, but equal in term, to that of the paternal figure. Partners who share children with incarcerated men become sole guardians, sole providers, and sole supporters of their children; they are inadvertently abandoned by their coparent and, therefore, left with no choice but to put other aspects of their life on hold. Aspects of which include those related to establishing a career, pursuing employment or educational opportunities, as well as those that include experiences offering the development and growth of qualities and attributes both personal and social in nature.

But if it were not for the children whom these parents share together, these two individuals would likely not find themselves in such a conflictual predicament in the first place, for it is a mutual desire to ensure the well-being of their children that binds them (whether complemented by a romantic attachment or not) and, in whose absence, a complete separation between the partners would be that much more likely. As such, the care and the well-being of the children remain the paramount focus. But if ensuring this well-being comes at the cost of one's freedom, in that it prevents them from pursuing other ventures, which of the two parents is more obligated to sacrifice this freedom, and which is more entitled to benefit from the relinquishment of such obligations?

Case Illustration: Jeremiah and Samantha

The case study of Jeremiah and Samantha reflects the conflicts that can arise when negotiating the roles and responsibilities of coparenting, both during incarceration and in the post-release period. Jeremiah is a 28-year-old African American male who shares a 2-year-old son with his long-time girlfriend, 27-year-old, White, female, Samantha. One year ago, Jeremiah was sentenced to nine months in a state penitentiary for third-degree assault, after a fight broke out at a local bar and in the process, Jeremiah severely injured the other person involved in the altercation. Jeremiah and Samantha debated whether Jeremiah should accept the nine-month sentence or opt for the three years of probation that the judge offered him as an alternative. Jeremiah previously had no criminal record, and the circumstances surrounding the altercation could not place the blame solely on Jeremiah. However, given the extent to which the other person involved was injured, Jeremiah was held completely liable.

Prior to Jeremiah's sentencing, he worked loading packages overnight for a large national carrier company, while Samantha was employed as a certified nursing assistant (CNA) during the day, while also in the process of exploring options to attend nursing school. Jeremiah was responsible for caring for their then infant son while Samantha was at work, and Samantha tended to the child at night during Jeremiah's shift. Although Jeremiah's incarceration would bring about a need for childcare, as well as eliminate one of the family's sources of income, the terms of Jeremiah's probation would require a 9 pm curfew, preventing him from working the night shift, which would in turn reduce his hourly wage significantly due to the differential he was currently being paid for working at night. Furthermore, Jeremiah's employer would be unable to offer him a dayshift for the foreseeable future due to their no existing openings at that time. They did, however, offer him his job back after he completed his sentence should a position be available. Samantha had apprehensions, although, recognizing that there was no good option, and that it was ultimately Jeremiah's decision, she eventually supported Jeremiah when he chose to accept the nine-month sentence.

While incarcerated, Samantha began working the night shift where she was employed, as this provided her with a wage increase – to offset the loss of Jeremiah's income – and she was able to rely on a combination of her and Jeremiah's relatives to watch their son at night. Within a month of this arrangement being established, it became apparent that the relatives who had offered their support would be unable to fulfill this responsibility reliably and consistently, and Samantha began to frequently miss shifts when no one was available to watch over the child. Samantha's employer was sympathetic initially and did not take any punitive measures. They ultimately offered Samantha an opportunity to return to the dayshift, which she accepted, but the reduction in wages rendered her unable to cover the costs of paid childcare without relying on a modest, but not insignificant amount of money that she had been saving to go toward nursing school. When this money ran out, and unable to afford childcare, Samantha had no choice but to resign from her job, at which point, she then qualified for public assistance, something she had previously been ineligible for due to the money she had held in savings.

When Jeremiah was eventually released, Samantha was relieved for a return to (perceived) normalcy. However, there were no open positions available at Jeremiah's former employer, whether during the day or at night. Therefore, having struggled so long financially, essentially as a single parent, she recognized how important it now was to her that she finally pursue her nursing degree, as the salary a nursing position would provide her with would ensure the family would never struggle again. Given that Jeremiah would be without a job anyway, at least at first, she wished to again begin working night shifts at her former employer, who was allowing her to return, to build back up the savings she had depleted while Jeremiah was incarcerated. Once she had done so, she planned to enroll in school, take day classes, and continue working night shifts as a CNA. In the meantime, Jeremiah would assume childcare duties until either a dayshift became available at his former employer, or he was able to obtain alternative employment elsewhere. Jeremiah initially agreed to this plan, as he recognized that, without a job immediately upon release, he would after all be home all day anyway. Samantha resumed working at night, while Jeremiah began looking for employment.

Initially, Jeremiah found himself unable to obtain an interview with any employers, until he finally was granted one after several weeks of searching. Instead of going to bed when she returned home from work that morning, Samantha stayed awake to keep an eye on their son while Jeremiah attended the job interview. Jeremiah was ecstatic when he returned home after the interview, sharing with Samantha that they had offered him the position. However, the shift would overlap with Samantha's and would require her to return to working during the day. This would increase their current income, however, because the pay they were offering him was significantly less than what he was making at his previous employer, and because Samantha's salary would decrease if she returned to working during the day, that increase would only be marginal.

Having put her dreams of attending nursing school on hold, and having struggled financially while Jeremiah was incarcerated, Samantha was adamant that they continue with their original plan and that Jeremiah simply continue seeking employment that would not disrupt their routine. However, not only was Jeremiah focused primarily on the current state of their finances, as opposed to Samantha, who was thinking about their future financial stability, Jeremiah had also been bottling up feelings of insecurity, inadequacy, and shame since the time he had been released. In a subsequent argument over how the family should proceed, Jeremiah snapped, and out of frustration exclaimed that he was "tired of being a stay-at-home mom!" and he was "tired of being trapped in the house all day, after being trapped in a jail cell for nine months!" Jeremiah wanted to work, he couldn't understand why Samantha wouldn't let him.

Samantha was livid, for having been, not a "stay-at-home mom" for the second half of Jeremiah's incarceration, but for having, instead, been an unemployed, single parent. Jeremiah's comment brought to the surface a previously nonexistent resentment against Jeremiah, given it was his actions that put her in that position. Until then, Samantha had been understanding and forgiving of Jeremiah. Furthermore, Samantha was offended that Jeremiah would express his frustration in that way, finding it sexist and unfair that the assumption was that child care should by default be the responsibility of the mother. Had he said, "stay-at-home dad", although still presumptuous, her reaction may not have been as drastic. Samantha felt that Jeremiah's ego and insecurity should not be prioritized over her aspirations, even if it meant a temporary alleviation of their financial difficulties, when the prospect of another solution becoming available, should Jeremiah hold off a little longer and continue seeking daytime employment, was very realistic.

An MFT could be helpful in resolving these disagreements by helping to ensure partner responsiveness to the wounded partner(s)'s emotional pain and attachment discomfort, which would help to alleviate the bond's rupture and encourage forgiveness and reconciliation (Zuccarini et al., 2013). It could also ensure new cycles of emotional engagement related to the injury to promote greater trust, relationship satisfaction, and forgiveness in resolved partners (Zuccarini et al., 2013). MFTs can also access the resiliency that comes with ensuring that a significant partner – in this case, Samantha or Jeremiah – will still be present and receptive.

Damaged Trust and the Need to Repair It

It is not uncommon for female caregivers to feel apprehensive about allowing the recently released father to spend time with the children alone, due to a lack of trust in their ability to safely supervise the children and out of fear that the children may be exposed to people or situations that could put them in harm's way. This is even more prominently the case when the mother is fully aware that the coparent has reestablished the same affiliations he had prior to incarceration, affiliations that previously brought with them criminal activities, which oftentimes led to the initial incarceration itself (Harman et al., 2007).

Research has demonstrated that in cases of coparenting, mothers do sometimes limit the amount of contact that fathers have with their children when risk factors are present or when the father's ability to parent effectively is questionable (Waller & Swisher, 2006). Consequently, the extent to which recently incarcerated fathers are involved in their children's lives post-release is limited when a significant level of mistrust in the father and a lack of confidence in his ability to safely and appropriately care for and supervise their children is possessed by the mother (Turney & Wildeman,

2013). Turney and Wildeman (2013) distinguish the actions of mothers in these instances from what is traditionally referred to as "gatekeeping". Gatekeeping, they identify, is a relational dynamic in which the power and control the father possesses, as they can be exercised in pursuit of seeing or speaking to his children, is significantly less, in some instances to the point of being completely nonexistent, than that which the mother possesses, as she can exercise them in either granting the father contact or communication with their children or not. Many factors outside the control of both parents – such as an incarceration facility's policies and access to resources – affect the degree of power both parents possess in this dynamic, while many factors may influence a mother's decision on how to exercise whatever degree of power she does possess; all of which are factors to be considered in a later section. However, in contrast, what Turney and Wildeman (2013) describe is better understood to be a protective measure taken by the mother out of caution and of an inadequate level of trust in the father, for the sole purpose of ensuring the children's safety.

This differentiation suggests that, in some cases, if a sufficient level of trust can be established between the coparents, then formerly incarcerated fathers very well could have an easier time establishing a meaningful level of involvement in their children's lives than might be so in coparenting relationships governed by a gatekeeping dynamic, and as a result, those barriers to a father's contact and communication with his children which arise out of the mother's apprehensions and concerns, could be overcome. In such a scenario, the father actually possesses a considerably greater degree of power than it may outwardly appear, given that the level of safety and security the father can provide to his children is directly impacted by–although not the only factor – decisions that only the father himself can make. Navigating such a scenario would require a willingness on the part of both parents to communicate and collaborate with one another respectfully and with graciousness and understanding, a process that could be facilitated by an MFT using relational therapy (Tadros, 2024).

Instances in which there are no safety concerns, or in those when the mother would withhold the children from the father even if there were not concerns, mothers often still possess, and take advantage of, the ability to limit or prevent contact. These instances will be understood to meet the definition of gatekeeping. This phenomenon often occurs while the father is currently incarcerated, but can also continue after his release, sustained for a variety of reasons and carried out for a multitude of motives, creating an additional barrier to the coparenting relationship and to be explored now.

Gatekeeping

While this section will focus primarily on situations in which gatekeeping occurs after a father is released from a correctional facility, it must be acknowledged that these situations likely did not begin at the onset of the post-release period but began while the father was still behind bars. The presence of this relational dynamic is simply more likely to be present during the incarceration period, given that the father possesses no power nor ability to see their children, independent of a reliance on a child's then current caregiver. Therefore, the occurrence of gatekeeping during the incarceration period will first be explored, before the presence of gatekeeping during the post-release period is then considered.

Often, the ones serving as guardians, and therefore as "gatekeepers"; non-incarcerated parents determine whether, and if so, how frequently, visitation or other forms of communication with an incarcerated father is beneficial to the child (Roy & Dyson, 2005; Tasca, 2016). Recent research on an enhanced visiting program implemented in a jail provides some insight into the prevalence of gatekeeping, revealing that only half of the children's caregivers were willing to participate in the intervention study (Charles et al., 2021). Many caregivers had negative feelings toward the incarcerated parent and were reluctant to make contact, while others were willing to allow the children to maintain contact despite their own reservations (Poehlmann-Tynan et al., 2015). It must be considered, however, that many caregivers were difficult to reach due to frequent relocations and changing phone numbers, a result of the economic challenges and residential instability common in families experiencing parental incarceration (Poehlmann-Tynan et al., 2015).

While these caregivers may have, under other circumstances, willingly participated, it must nonetheless be noted that increased efforts on the part of the caregiver to remain in contact with the incarcerated parent, despite changing residences or means of communication, may have overcome this barrier. This inadequate level of effort could be explained in two different ways, either that:

1 Caregivers do not always prioritize ensuring that contact between incarcerated parents and their children occurs, by reporting to the correctional facility changes in residence or telephone numbers, which could be considered, to some extent, a form of gatekeeping.
2 The effects of incarceration, exacerbated by current policy, impact the families of incarcerated individuals to the extent that ensuring this contact occurs is excessively challenging.

Either scenario is problematic, both so for a variety of reasons. Given caregivers' role as gatekeepers, fostering more positive coparenting relationships could increase opportunities for parent-child contact, leading to improved parent-child relationships and child well-being.

Given that an increased level of contact and connections between incarcerated parents and their children produces more positive outcomes related to childhood development, as well as improves parent-child relationships – two domains detrimentally affected by parental incarceration, both during and after the incarceration period – a reduction in the prevalence of gatekeeping during the incarceration period should be a priority by policymakers and clinicians. Consequently, such research draws into question whether caregivers, despite being those who decide whether and how frequent contact occurs, may in fact not always know what is most beneficial to the child.

On a broader scale, independent of but in addition to the presence of gatekeeping, several other factors hinder the strengthening of coparenting and overall family bonds during incarceration. Mediations that encourage incarcerated fathers to engage in open discussions about their background, upbringing, and relationship with the children's mother can facilitate a smoother reintegration into the family home. Such interventions give way to an exploration of the presence of gatekeeping during the post-release period, the emphasis of this chapter. What factors sustain such an arrangement once the obvious barriers, exacerbated by incarceration, have fallen away?

To begin to attempt to answer this question, one must consider the obvious, which is that, if a precedent of gatekeeping has occurred during the incarceration period, then why might one expect this tendency to immediately dissipate as soon as the incarceration period has ended? One shouldn't. Although many of the structural factors erected and supported by the policies and facilities that define and carry out incarceration in the United States may have fallen away, the desires of some non-incarcerated coparents to continue withholding contact between now recently released fathers from their jointly shared child(ren) remain. It's worthy of exploring the reasons that this desire remains as well as what circumstantially as well as institutional factors may encourage or, at least, support it.

Although some coparenting arrangements involve married individuals, more often than not, unmarried fathers and mothers share in the coparenting arrangement and do so as a result of a naturally occurring arrangement precipitated by their shared children. However, despite this mutual reliance existing in the interest of the children prior to the incarceration period, such an arrangement has been sustained independent of legal or custodial agreements. Upon release, previously incarcerated men find themselves without any sort of legal support, adrift without any form of custodial guarantees, yet desiring a relationship with their children. Meanwhile, the mother has taken upon herself full responsibility for the well-being of the shared children during the incarceration, creating a scenario in which, should custodial or visitation arrangements be sought on the part of the recently released father, the courts would likely side on her behalf.

Attempts for equitable custodial arrangements, quite possibly even simply established visitation arrangements, made on the part of the father, should he even have the resources and possess the wherewithal to pursue such an end, would likely see the courts side overwhelmingly on behalf of the mother, and understandably so. Was she not solely responsible for the well-being of the child(ren) during the incarceration period? And considering his criminal record, what court would deem him even an equal, let alone a superior, caregiver compared to the mother?

And there do not exist any shortage of reasons why the mother may choose to withhold contact between the shared children and the recently released coparent. As previously explored, there exist a multitude of reasons that the coparent of an incarcerated father may have developed resentments against him, for the perceived abandonment his incarceration has caused her and any shared children, the financial hardship that she encountered as a result, and for possible infidelity which may have arisen since he has been released, among others. It should come as no surprise that the female coparent may choose to withhold contact between the shared child(ren) and the recently released father, if not only because it allows her to avoid interactions with him, and not even necessarily because she is motivated solely by a desire to prevent contact between father and child(ren). Considering this, it would not be unreasonable to draw the conclusion that the mother of shared children may also struggle to see the father as a father, in the fullest capacity of the word, therefore, feeling as though efforts made on her part to ensure regular father-child contact post-release is not something the father is deserving of. It could even be the case that it is not only efforts to ensure contact are not made, but that a deliberate and intentional withholding of contact occurs. Mothers of shared children could conceivably view father-child contact as a privilege and not a right, and therefore until this privilege is earned, the presence of gatekeeping will persist.

Furthermore, recently released fathers must navigate their coparenting partner's new partner at times, scenarios sometimes arising in which the mother of his child(ren) has entered into a romantic relationship with another man during his incarceration and one who has assumed, to varying degrees, the role of "stepfather". A two-parent household has been created in the father's absence and the father's release may, understandably so, but at the very least in the eyes of the mother, serve to disrupt the stability that has been attained in his absence. Actions could very well be taken to keep the recently released father from suddenly disrupting such stability.

What's a Father to Do?

As discussed in previous chapters, many barriers to regular contact and communication between incarcerated individuals and their loved ones exist, and relationships suffer as a result. Nonetheless, mending and reestablishing an adult relationship post-release can and does occur, especially made easier when that relationship had already existed for an extended period of time prior to incarceration. However, in the case of incarcerated parents and their children, reuniting after having been apart for a period of time is less predictable. Depending on the duration of one's sentence, the age of the child at the time of incarceration, and the amount of contact that occurred between parent and child during incarceration, it may be the case that the relationship does not in fact need to be mended or reestablished at all, but instead, established for the very first time altogether.

Likewise, while an incarcerated individual may feel guilty for the burden that has been placed on their romantic partner while they were away, as was explored in the previous chapter, the inadequacies with which a parent identifies for being absent in their child's life due to their incarceration are quite debilitating themselves (Tripp, 2001). These factors influence the role that formerly incarcerated fathers take on after they have been released, defining how they come to parent their children. At times, the way they fulfill this parental role, uniquely influenced by their incarceration, can conflict with the second caregiver's approach to raising shared children, generating discord in the coparenting relationship (Visher & Travis, 2003). Before exploring the nature of this discord, it is important to gain an understanding of how incarcerated men experience this separation from their children.

Hairston (1998) draws a distinction between what she calls the "prevailing view" of who incarcerated fathers are – with particular focus on African American fathers – and who they are in truth (p. 620). Hairston identifies a widely held perception of these men, one which characterizes them as being absent as fathers prior to their incarceration as inaccurate and, in contestation, proposes that their fulfillment of the paternal role may in fact simply look different from that with which those who hold this misperception are familiar. Although the quaint and idyllic picture of the traditional nuclear family – one comprised of husband, wife, and children, all biologically related, and long a figment of middle America's collective imagination – would not bear any superficial resemblance to the household compositions of which incarcerated fathers are or were formerly members, many of whom share children with multiple women, and with whom they were never married, most of these fathers did in fact live in the same household as at least one of their children immediately preceding their incarceration. More importantly however, many of these men shared strong emotional attachments with their children, while providing care to them physically, even when they could not necessarily do so financially, and actively spending time with them. Incarceration, however, disrupts these relationships, stunting the natural progression of their development and sometimes preventing it altogether.

The emotional impact of this consequence on incarcerated fathers, as well as on their perceptions of themselves, should not be understated. Through conducting multiple interviews and focus groups involving 12 incarcerated African American fathers, as part of a wider prison program devoted to the development of "life skills", Tripp (2001) identified two, of what he refers to as, *orientations* that informed these men's understanding of fatherhood: *action orientation* and *child orientation*. He then reported on the men's experiences attempting to, sometimes successfully but more often not, live up to these understandings.

Those fathers who were identified as possessing an *action orientation* placed value in the actions taken by a father in his children's lives, viewing them as indicators of the quality with which he is fulfilling the role of father. Some of the actions shared by participants included such things as assisting with homework, treating the children to food or activities, and spending time with them. Additionally, less tangible actions were offered as examples, including providing things such as guidance and discipline. These men placed a notable emphasis on the importance of a father's physical presence in the home when raising children (Tripp, 2001).

In contrast, fathers more closely aligned with a *child orientation* in how they understood fatherhood, determined one's quality as a father based on the child's behavior and the characteristics present in the father-child relationship. Men of this orientation considered themselves good fathers if, for example, their children were well-behaved, performed well in school, trusted them as guardians, and respected them. If these qualities were not present in their children, these men believed that they had not fulfilled their paternal responsibility successfully and were therefore not good fathers (Tripp, 2001).

As men who, prior to their incarceration, according to Hairston (1998), placed value in the relationships they shared with their children as well as in fulfilling their paternal responsibilities, the obvious barriers that incarceration presents in continuing to do so have a damaging impact on their own self-perception. Tripp (2001) notes that some of the participants struggled to even identify themselves as fathers, given that incarceration prevented them from being physically present for their children, participating in activities with them, providing material things to them as well as limited their ability to offer guidance, instill discipline, and serve as positive role models; as ones who might encourage the development of positive qualities in their children's character. Additionally, when these men talked of their children developing problematic behaviors in the time since their incarceration, a common consequence of paternal incarceration (Giordano et al., 2019), they held themselves, for not being present, wholly responsible (Tripp, 2001). Many children do indeed experience adverse effects due to their parent's incarceration, including the stigma associated with being a child whose parent is incarcerated and the trauma that incarceration may inflict on him or her, which can play out as behavioral issues. The children also may experience secondary impacts of incarceration from their parents being affected by their incarceration, which, in turn, impacts their ability to parent the child.

When released, formerly incarcerated fathers must now encounter and engage with any potential fallout, whether internal to them or found in their interactions with their children, that exists as a result of their absence. Many continue to report a desire to be directly involved in their children's lives and seek to achieve this through engaging in recreational activities as the method by which they might form or mend relationships with them.

Paradoxically, they simultaneously report feeling discomfort at this prospect – earning credit where they believe no credit is due – given that they struggle to provide for the family in other ways, for instance, financially. Feeling as though they lack credibility as men and as fathers, both due to their previous absence and to the limited ways in which they are able to provide practical support to their families, some fathers experience inner conflict, as they attempt to locate their role within the family and within the coparenting arrangement. It is not unusual that this leads fathers to tilt more in the direction of being a "friend" to their children than of a "parent" (Harman et al., 2007) due to their ability to create a "fun" environment in the face of their inability to provide a structured one. Concerned with external and internal perceptions of credibility as fathers, as providers, protectors, and role models, having been absent in these roles for so long, men may discover that pursuing a relationship with their children characterized more so by the presence of agreeability, humor, and enjoyment, rather than by the presence of qualities such as stability, authoritativeness, respect, and dependability, is the more assured approach to establishing themselves as important persons in their children's lives.

It has previously been noted that one of the consequences of incarceration is the emergence of behavioral issues among children (Giordano et al., 2019). However, even in cases where the previously incarcerated father is willing to take on a more traditionally paternal role, they are limited in the ways they can address behavioral issues, due to the resistance the coparent has toward the father disciplining or reprimanding the child, frequently being interrupted or diverted by the coparent when attempts to do so are made (Harman et al., 2007). Mothers may not feel as though the father is deserving of the authority necessary to discipline a child, given their prolonged absence and the hardship the family experienced as a result.

Women who have adjusted to the release from prison of their children's father and have experienced the process of reintegrating them into their own and their children's lives in a useful and contributory way, when interviewed, have often identified themselves as ones who relate to their children as being more akin to friends or older siblings than as parents. They have elaborated that the possibility of this role of "friend" evolving into one more traditionally paternal in nature remains contingent upon the mother's own discretion and influenced by the length of time that the man has remained out of prison (Harman et al., 2007). Consequently, the inadequacy that men feel in assuming the more traditionally paternalistic qualities as fathers – such as disciplinarian and provider – find it complemented and affirmed through the aforementioned position of the coparent.

However, should the previously incarcerated father, upon release, reinitiate himself in his children's lives by assuming the role of "friend", "buddy", or "pal", for the purpose of developing and maintaining a bond with his children by any feasible means necessary, it may cause a disruption in the children and mother's lives, by serving as an interruption of and detraction away from how the mother has managed to maintain a household and raise her children effectively, absent a paternal figure, by acting too leniently in regards to discipline and privileges. Were a child to "misbehave" and thus be subject to discipline by the coparenting mother, the recently released father may attempt to circumvent this discipline to strengthen the relationship the two feel together.

If they attempt to assume the role of "head of household", they feel presumptuous, phony, undeserving or lacking in credibility, while facing resistance from the coparent. But if they assume the role of friend, for the purpose of establishing a relationship – given the insecurities and inadequacies they possess, along with resistance from the mother – they run the risk of undermining the routine and authority of, as well as the expectations set by, the coparenting mother during the time of their incarceration. Meanwhile, this paradox may further conflict with expectations that coparents have for the father to assume the role of supervisor and caretaker of the children, as discussed in a previous section, allowing the mother to resume employment and other engagements.

If a father wishes to be more than just a friend, he must gain credibility as a provider, for instance, through obtaining employment. He may find himself unable to do so if he is assigned childcare duties. And yet, with what authority and credibility does he possess the ability to make decisions affecting the child regarding offering privileges and implementing discipline while supervising them? If he does not assume the role of supervisor appropriately, he may never shed the role of friend, but if he assumes the role of disciplinarian too liberally, he may be dissuaded to do anything but continue behaving as a friend. So, what's a father to do?

References

Charles, P., Kerr, M., Wirth, J., Jensen, S., Massoglia, M., & Poehlmann-Tynan, J. (2021). Lessons from the field: Developing and implementing an intervention for jailed parents and their children. *Family Relations*, *70*(1), 171–178. https://doi.org/10.1111/fare.12524

Comfort, M., Krieger, K. E., Landwehr, J., McKay, T., Lindquist, C. H., Feinberg, R., Kennedy, E. K., & Bir, A. (2018). Partnership after prison: Couple relationships during reentry. *Journal of Offender Rehabilitation*, *57*(2), 188–205. https://doi.org/10.1080/10509674.2018.1441208

Ghandnoosh, N., Stammen, E., & Muhitch, K. *Parents in prison*. The Sentencing Project. https://www.sentencingproject.org/policy-brief/parents-in-prison/

Giordano, P. C., Copp, J. E., Manning, W. D., & Longmore, M. A. (2019). Linking parental incarceration and family dynamics associated with intergenerational transmission: A life course perspective. *Criminology*, *57*, 395–423. https://doi.org/10.1111/1745-9125.12209

Hairston, C. F. (1998). The forgotten parent: Understanding the forces that influence incarcerated fathers' relationships with their children. *Child Welfare*, *77*(5), 617–639. https://www.jstor.org/stable/45400149

Harman, J. J., Smith, V. E., & Egan, L. C. (2007). The impact of incarceration on intimate relationships. *Criminal Justice and Behavior*, *34*(6), 794–815.https://doi.org/10.1177/0093854807299543

Poehlmann-Tynan, J., Runion, H., Burnson, C., Maleck, S., Weymouth, L., Pettit, K., & Huser, M. (2015). Young children's behavioral and emotional reactions to plexiglas and video visits with jailed parents. In *Children's contact with incarcerated parents: Implications for policy and intervention* (pp. 39–58). Springer International Publishing, Cham, Switzerland. https://doi.org/10.1007/978-3-319-16625-4_3

Roy, K. M., & Dyson, O. L. (2005). Gatekeeping in context: Babymama drama and the involvement of incarcerated fathers. *Fathering: A Journal of Theory, Research, and Practice About Men As Fathers*, *3*(3), 289–310.

Tadros, E. (2024). The importance of the 'village': Examining social supports and hazardous alcohol use among mothers with an incarcerated coparent. *American Journal of Family Therapy*, *52*(1), 1–21. https://doi.org/10.1080/01926187.2022.2040400

Tasca, M. (2016). The gatekeepers of contact: Child–caregiver dyads and parental prison visitation. *Criminal Justice and Behavior*, *43*(6), 739–758. https://doi.org/10.1177/0093854815613528

Tripp, B. (2001). Incarcerated African American fathers: Exploring changes in family relationships and the father identity. *Journal of African American Men*, *6*(1), 13–29. https://doi.org/10.1007/s12111-001-1011-5

Turney, K., & Wildeman, C. (2013). Redefining relationships: Explaining the countervailing consequences of paternal incarceration for parenting. *American Sociological Review*, *78*(6), 949–979. https://doi.org/10.1177/0003122413505589

Visher, C. A., & Travis, J. (2003). Transitions from prison to community: Understanding individual pathways. *Annual Review of Sociology*, *29*, 89–113. https://doi.org/10.1146/annurev.soc.29.010202.100009

Waller, M. R., & Swisher, R. (2006). Fathers' risk factors in fragile families: Implications for "healthy" relationships and father involvement. *Social Problems*, *53*(3), 392–420. https://doi.org/10.1525/sp.2006.53.3.392

Zuccarini, D., Johnson, S. M., Dalgleish, T. L., & Makinen, J. A. (2013). Forgiveness and reconciliation in emotionally focused therapy for couples: The client change process and therapist interventions. *Journal of Marital and Family Therapy*, *39*(2), 148–162. https://doi.org/10.1111/j.1752-0606.2012.00287.x

Chapter 11

Future Research and Policy Directions

Shawn Wunderlich

Future Research and Advocacy Directions

Further research needs to be conducted on family therapy and incarcerated individuals. Currently, most of the research is focused on juveniles and the incarcerated individual with little studies done on incarcerated mothers, family members, and post-release therapeutic intervention (Tadros et al., 2024). While much of the research does focus on juveniles, there are very few studies conducted on adults in the United States who have had a child become incarcerated (Tadros et al., 2025). Two recent studies focus on adults who have the experience of having an adult child incarcerated (Tadros et al., 2024; Tadros et al., 2025). Further, very little studies have been done on incarcerated mothers, family members, and post-therapeutic interventions as well as community support strategies. This severely limits the ability to further understand the needs of this population thus severely limiting the ability to create programs and treatment modalities to help support these individuals.

In the context of relationships, current studies focus on the incarcerated individual and their non-offending partner. The context of these studies focuses on improving communication, regulation, and relationship satisfaction (Kazura, 2018). Future research should be conducted on the non-prison partner and what their expectations of the incarcerated individual are upon release, in terms of being a couple or in the family. If non-incarcerated partners have certain expectations that cannot be fulfilled right away by the incarcerated partner, further education should be done on what to expect upon release. This can lower expectations which can set the family up for success and less conflict. Additionally, it may be important for the non-incarcerated partner to learn how to communicate their expectations and needs to their incarcerated partner to further improve communication and understanding of how their family culture will operate.

While it is important to understand the partner's expectations and roles in the post release of the incarcerated partner, it is also important to study

DOI: 10.4324/9781003542940-11

how communities respond to an individual who has been incarcerated. Specifically, it would be important to learn what types of resources are available, if the individual has utilized them or knows about them, and what the viewpoint is in the community regarding incarcerated individuals. It would be worth understanding if there is a stigma in the community and what that stigma "says". This type of study could impact the individual in that workshops and educational groups can be created and present information regarding supporting incarcerated individuals. This may pave the way to additional resources in communities and change in policy around post-release work, support, etc.

Beyond the non-offending partner and community, studies should also focus on incarcerated mothers. Currently, most research is done on males, but mothers are also incarcerated and bring about unique challenges and needs than those of their counterpart. A study conducted on being a mother post release could benefit not only the mother but also the children. It would be important to learn more about how society can support mothers in prison settings, what the impact is for the mother and child during and post release, and what types of interventions and resources are currently available for mothers during and post release. These studies would significantly benefit these individuals in that programs can be created that can be focused only on mothers who are incarcerated. The results of the study can also impact the children in that a program can be created to help support both children and mother. Furthermore, policy can be changed that can require additional support for mothers and their children with more visits, communication, and bonding time between child and mother.

While research has currently focused on specific interventions that can help contribute to successful relationships post release, it would also be important to study if there are any specific family conflicts that occur most often. This would help with the creation of programs that can focus on the most common experiences as it relates to family conflict. Additionally, studying health family functioning post release can pave way to additional information on the needs of those incarcerated and their partners. It would be beneficial to learn more about healthy functioning post release so that programs and interventions can be created to promote healthy functioning post release. Studies can focus on resilience and strength in families that have healthy functioning post release so that a focus can occur on these characteristics while the individual is in prison.

Studies have also focused on specific programs, like the prevention and relationship enhancement program, and how these have impacted the incarcerated individual's relationship, from the viewpoint of the incarcerated individual and their partner (Kazura, 2018). It would be beneficial to assess the family members' involvement and outcomes from their perspective. Do family members feel there is a chance within the relationship and if so, how? How do family members experience the relationship during and post incarceration with the incarcerated individual? Gaining further understanding of how the family members experience the relationship with the incarcerated individual will assist therapists, community members, and the like to create additional interventions, programs, and policy. If the interventions have been deemed helpful in promoting a positive relationship between the incarcerated individual and the family member, there should be a push to utilize these interventions across all who are incarcerated. This will further assist the individual in maintaining social support and gaining additional support post-incarceration thus potentially limiting recidivism. Additionally, a study that follows a family over time would be helpful in learning how these interventions and programs last over time to further provide evidence for the implementation of these interventions across all who are incarcerated.

Further, trauma is prevalent not only pre-incarceration but also during incarceration. Additionally, trauma can occur post incarceration when the incarcerated individual is released. Depending on how long the individual has been away from their family and incarcerated, there could have been many societal changes that have occurred thus making it harder for the individual to adjust to post-incarceration life. This can be traumatic in itself, on top of the loss of family members and friends who may have passed while in prison. This loss can contribute to significant trauma and shame. Thus, it would be incredibly important to study trauma and incarcerated individuals. It would be important to learn more about the incarceration experience and how this impacts the individual post-release. Learning about the trauma incarcerated individuals may experience post-release can also be beneficial in creating programs to prepare the individual prior to being released. Not only is it important to study the trauma experienced by the incarcerated individual, it is also important to learn more about the trauma that the family may experience. The results of a study such as this would help program implementation and interventions for the family to decrease the possibility of intergenerational trauma that can and does occur.

Finally, most of the research is being conducted on individuals who have already been incarcerated which allows programs to be implemented for the prison setting. It would actually be important for research to be conducted for the purpose of prevention. If researchers can learn more about what, within the family, may have led to incarceration, how the individual experiences the family during and post incarceration, and what tools can be utilized. Additional programs can be developed to support at-risk individuals, helping to prevent initial offenses or reduce the likelihood of reoffending.

Call to Action

Advocacy in the mental health profession began more than 30 years ago and was developed to promote the human rights of those suffering from mental illness (Levin, 2019). It also promotes change to reduce the stigma and discrimination of these individuals by utilizing various actions to change major structural and attitudinal barriers (Saha, 2021). Furthermore, advocacy is one of the 11 areas for action in mental health policy due to the benefits it has for those with mental health disorders and their families (Saha, 2021). One of the biggest reasons for advocacy is the need for reduction of stigma and a change in policy and legislation. The incarcerated population needs to be advocated for now more than ever.

Stigma Associated with Incarceration

Before a discussion occurs on how to advocate for this population, it is important to call out the stigma that these individuals face within their communities, families, and within themselves and discuss how communities specifically can assist de-stigmatization. The stigma of being an incarcerated individual is so prevalent that criminology theories have been created to explain this phenomenon. Labeling theory is one theoretical perspective that has been discussed in literature, and it identifies that being labeled as an "offender" causes the individual to internalize stigmatizing attitudes, withdraw from society and conform to a deviant identity (Lemert, 1974). Stigma affects an individual in many ways. Link and Phelan (2001), outline three factors of stigma: structural (i.e. interactions among institutional barriers), social (i.e. stereotypes and discrimination from community members), and self (i.e. perception of self). Communities can directly impact all three of these factors of stigma. They can create institutional barriers and perpetuate stereotypes by not working alongside the incarcerated individual, both of which can further perpetuate the self-stigma these individuals may have. Additionally, it is important to note two types of stigma that can occur: anticipated stigma (i.e. expectation of personally experiencing discrimination due to having a stigmatized identity, Winnick & Bodkin, 2008) and perceived stigma (i.e. perceptions that society holds negative views of a group and what someone may experience as a result of stigma, (Major & Sawyer, 2009) with incarcerated individuals. Both of these types of stigma can result in behaviors that can cause further harm to the individual.

While the rest of the chapter will discuss ways in which correctional administrators and community members can help those who have been incarcerated, it is also important to identify ways in which community members can de-stigmatize incarceration, specifically due to the fact that they can directly influence all three factors of stigma and are likely the first experience the incarcerated individual has upon reentry.

Firstly, it is important for these individuals to receive counseling services to assist in self-stigma. Exploring their perceptions of their incarceration experience and working on addressing any negative perceptions of self can be incredibly beneficial to the individual in reducing shame and negative self-concept. This can reduce negative behaviors that can result from self-stigma. It is also important to educate the community about the stigma of incarceration. It is important to highlight reasons why one might commit a crime and address the systemic disparities that might influence incarceration (i.e. social, racial/ethnic, mental health, and housing). While further discussion on how community members can help those who have been incarcerated will be discussed in full later, it is important to make note that the community can have a direct impact in the stigmatization of those who have been incarcerated.

Communities have a shared responsibility to support those who have been incarcerated because, ultimately, they come from the same place. Listening to their voice is crucial in understanding the unique challenges they face and what they need to successfully enter back into society. Those who have been incarcerated are not only isolated from the community they came from, they also witness or experience violence in correctional facilities, face isolation, and lose many basic rights. When these individuals return to their community, they may encounter further obstacles like isolation from their community, finding stable work, resolving conflict in healthy ways, and managing mental health challenges that they may have developed due to being incarcerated. The stigma points to these individuals as untrustworthy or irredeemable, which only exacerbates these struggles, reinforces their negative beliefs about themselves, and makes it harder to rebuild their lives. Rather than further alienating them, communities must recognize that these individuals' success is intertwined with the health of the broader society and supporting their transition is essential for creating safer, more inclusive environments for all.

Education is an incredibly powerful tool to support individuals who have been incarcerated. It allows communities to better understand complex factors that contribute to criminal behavior. By learning about the systemic disparities that often lead individuals to commit crimes, communities can gain insight into the root cause of incarceration. Education will shed light on the trauma, violence, and emotional pain these individuals may endure in prison, which may hinder successful reintegration. When communities have this knowledge, they can not only provide more effective support for those reentering society, but they can also advocate for systemic changes to address injustices that perpetuate the cycle of crime and incarceration. This will foster a more compassionate, proactive approach to preventing crime and promote healing for the individual and society.

Correctional Administrators

Five million youth experience parental incarceration before they reach age 18 (Murphey & Cooper, 2015). When children have an incarcerated parent, they are significantly more likely to experience homelessness, housing instability, food insecurity, and lower rates of educational achievement (Arabyan, 2022; Foster & Hagan, 2009; Johnson, 2009; Wakefield & Wildeman, 2014). Furthermore, children of incarcerated individuals have an increase in mental health issues and destabilization in the family unit (Sexton, 2016).

Due to the increased consequences for children of incarcerated individuals, it is important to advocate for changes within the prison settings so that children are experiencing less mental health issues. Arabyan (2022) found that children who have an incarcerated parent must change their lives and process the fact that their parent is incarcerated. It would be important to implement programs that specifically address children who have incarcerated family members. One way to do this would be to implement a program that children can attend, where they can work on processing the fact that their family member is in prison. It would utilize counseling techniques and interventions to allow children a safe place to voice what they feel and think about their family member being incarcerated. They would have a mental health therapist assigned to them where they can also utilize individual therapy to discuss more unique concerns of the child. They would also attend group therapy where they can connect with others who have a parent who is incarcerated.

Connection to family plays a role in recidivism rates and more visits to the incarcerated family member shows a decrease in recidivism rates (Greenwood, 2016). There is power in bringing family members together allowing for a greater awareness into how members contribute to the system in the family (Cammett et al., 2017). There is a need for change in the prison settings as it relates to family therapy, and I think those in the mental health field can work to advocate for this change.

Family therapy would benefit the family unit in processing through the experience of having an incarcerated family member. It can be utilized to empower caregivers to solve problems (Garofalo, 2020) and reduce family conflict (Garofalo, 2020). It improves family cohesion and support (Datchi et al., 2016). These outcomes can impact overall recidivism rates with a decrease occurring due to family therapy (Greenwood, 2016).

Prevention and relationship enhancement programs help reduce the negative impact of incarceration on families (Kazura, 2018), upon completing the program, incarcerated individuals and their partners found more positive interactions, a greater confidence in their relationship, and additional education regarding maintaining healthy relationships. If a parent goes through a prevention and relationship enhancement program, they learn the skills to improve their overall relationship with their partner which can trickle down into the family unit thus potentially lowering the possibility for their children to become incarcerated individuals in the future. It also helps lower the chance of recidivism because these individuals will have received adequate support and experienced better familial and relationship outcomes.

When looking at coparenting, there is often a strain on the non-offending parent as they are left with caretaking for children while the offending individual is incarcerated. This can create conflict within the couple which can impact the family unit. Children of parents who are incarcerated have an increased risk for developing behavioral problems, academic failure, and substance use (Poehlmann et al., 2010). Parent-child relationship is an important factor as it relates to later social and emotional functioning (Thompson, 2008), and attachment to caregivers is equally important whether the parent is incarcerated or at home (Poehlmann, 2005). This further identifies the importance of positive coparenting and the ability for connection between the caregiver who is incarcerated and the child. Arditti (2012) found that individuals may have difficulty coparenting, specifically when the father is incarcerated, specifically, incarcerated fathers had difficulty contacting children and relied on the biological mother for collaboration. Mothers may gatekeep which not only impacts the relationship with the mother and father but also impacts the relationship between father and child. The child's caregiver has more ability to control if the child gets a phone call or mail from the incarcerated parent and they are the individual who will determine if the child will be able to visit the incarcerated parent (Shlafer & Poelman, 2010). If a caregiver is gatekeeping a child, they are keeping the child away from the incarcerated parent which later impacts attachment and connection between the incarcerated parent and their child. The gatekeeping process will be influenced by the parent's relationship. If the relationship between the incarcerated parent and the non-incarcerated parent is dysfunctional, there may be a higher likelihood that visitation to the incarcerated parent will be limited. This can severely impact the child's relationship with their incarcerated parent (Johnson & Easterling, 2012) which increases the likelihood that the child becomes an incarcerated individual themselves thus contributing to intergenerational incarceration and trauma. It would be incredibly beneficial to advocate for programs to be created for non-prison partners and their family. It should focus on increasing communication, providing regular visits, and quality time between the incarcerated individual and their family members (Tadros et al., 2022, 2023).

Communities

A community can influence the likelihood of incarceration for its community members. A community that supports one another, creates and has opportunity, and has resources for its members could be beneficial for its members. Research has found various factors within communities that contribute to higher levels of incarceration, and it is important to work toward creating change that will positively impact the community members. Communities who have higher levels of poverty and unemployment as well as lower levels of education are often seeing higher levels of incarceration compared to other communities (Clear, 2007). If a community does not have the resources to assist its members, it may see higher levels of substance use and mental health issues, lower employment opportunities, and lower availability of affordable housing (Travis et al., 2001). Morenhoff and Harding (2014) report that many incarcerated individuals live alongside those who are formerly incarcerated post-release which may result in competition for already low resources thus the potential for reoffending occurs (Morenoff & Harding, 2014).

Additional research finds that incarceration can impact communities by creating a gender imbalance, lower quantity of male role models (Morenoff & Harding, 2014), lack of collectivism and increased social disorganization (Drakulich et al., 2012), weakened political power of low-income and minoritized communities (United States Commission on Civil Rights, 2019), and increased crime (Rose & Clear, 1998).

Creating community assistance is of the utmost importance in assisting incarcerated individuals re-integrate into society post release with a higher likelihood of reducing recidivism. It would be important for community members to secure resources and seek out additional support from neighboring communities. One way to create community support is through community engagement. Travis et al. (2001) recommend developing neighborhood-based networks or local businesses who will assist in preparing the incarcerated individual in securing employment post release, engaging community-based organizations to assist family members of incarcerated individuals so that the family can support a successful reentry. Additionally, involving local faith-based institutes for mentoring and providing the formerly incarcerated individual opportunities to participate in community services and further assist in feeling involved in a supportive network. Finally, develop a coalition of resident leaders to oversee these reentry efforts and make sure that the individual is getting the necessary resources that are available to them.

Behavioral health and the legal system are typically treated separately despite so many incarcerated individuals having mental health diagnoses. In fact, 45% of the jail population reported a history of mental health issues in 2017 (Bronson & Berzofsky, 2017), with the percentage of individuals meeting criteria for a serious mental health diagnosis (26%) being five times greater than the general population of non-incarcerated individuals (Bronson & Berzofsky, 2017). Because of this, it is important for community members to put effort into creating more behavioral health services to assist the community in ensuring early intervention as well as support for those who are already involved in the legal system. Some have argued that incarceration has taken the place of hospitalization since the 1960s (Wacquant, 2009). Those who suffer mental health issues who are incarcerated may experience additional mental health issues due to being incarcerated. Recent studies have estimated that as increases occur in incarceration, specifically in jails, the rate of county-wide mortality from substance use and suicide also increases (Kajeepeta et al., 2021). Many communities may not have the resources to focus on behavioral health care. Rural communities tend to have fewer mental health services (Thomas et al., 2009) and are less likely to accept Medicaid (Cummings et al., 2013). Communities that have higher Black and/or Hispanic populations have reduced access to behavioral services as well (Ellis et al., 2009). This severely limits the ability for community members to seek services before it is absolutely needed. It also restricts the options available to assist individuals who commit crimes (Fisher et al., 2006). Those who have mental health disorders who commit crimes may engage in criminal behavior due to poverty and unemployment, lack of housing, low self-control, and substance dependence (Lurigio, 2011). There have been many studies that have found that as services for higher levels of care decrease, incarceration rates increase (Gao, 2021).

Greater support is needed for incarcerated individuals during and after incarceration. This can help to reduce recidivism, address mental health needs, and support family reunification. Incarceration impacts individuals as well as families, especially children. Expanding counseling, social work, and family therapy programs focused on this population could improve outcomes, reduce trauma, and challenge systemic stigma. Society needs to advocate for this population and shift from turning away to leaning in with meaningful support.

References

Arabyan, K. (2022). "Adaptation program: Systemic treatment of incarcerated individuals and their families" Loma Linda University Electronic Theses, Dissertations & Projects. 1749. https://scholarsrepository.llu.edu/etd/1749

Arditti, J. A. (2012). *Parental incarceration and the family: Psychological and social effects of imprisonment on children, parents, and caregivers.* New York University Press.

Bronson, J., & Berzofsky, M. (2017). Indicators of mental health problems reported by prisoners and jail inmates, 2011–12. *Bureau of Justice Statistics*, 1–16. https://www.bjs.gov/content/pub/pdf/imhprpji1112.pdf

Cammett, A. (2017). Reflections on the challenge of Inez Moore: Family integrity in the wake of mass incarceration. *Fordham Law Review*, *85*(6), 2579–2587. https://ir.lawnet.fordham.edu/flr/vol85/iss6/5

Clear, T. R. (2007). *Imprisoning communities: How mass incarceration makes disadvantaged neighborhoods worse.* New York: Oxford Press.

Cummings, J. R., Wen, H., & Druss, B. G. (2013). Improving access to mental health services for youth in the United States. *JAMA, 309*(6), 553–554.

Datchi, C. C., Barretti, L. M., & Thompson, C. M. (2016). Family services in adult detention centers: Systemic principles for prisoner reentry. *Couple and Family Psychology: Research and Practice, 5*(2), 89–104. https://doi.org/10.1037/cfp0000057

Drakulich, K. M., Crutchfield, R. D., Matsueda, R. L., & Rose, K. (2012). Instability, informal social control, and crimogenic situations: Community effects of returning prisoners. *Crime, Law, and Social Change, 57*, 493–519.

Ellis, A. R., Konrad, T. R., Thomas, K. C., & Morrissey, J. P (2009). County-level estimates of mental health professional supply in the United States. *Psychiatric Services, 60*(1), 1315–1322. https://doi.org/10.1176/ps.2009.60.10.1315.

Fisher, W. H., Silver, K., & Wolff, N. (2006). Beyond criminalization: Towards criminologically informed framework for mental health policy and services research. *Administration and Policy in Mental Health and Mental Health Services, 33*(5), 544–557. https://doi.org/10.1007/s10488-006-0072-0

Foster, H., & Hagan, J. (2009). The mass incarceration of parents in America: Issues of race/ ethnicity, collateral damage to children, and prisoner reentry. *The Annals of the American Academy of Political and Social Science, 623*, 179–194. https://dx.doi.org/10.1177/0002716208331123

Garofalo, M. (2020) Family therapy in corrections: Implications for reentry into the community. *Journal of Correctional Health Care, 26*(3), 240–248. https://doi.org/10.1177/1078345820938350

Gao, Y. N. (2021). The relationship between psychiatric inpatient beds and jail populations in the United States. *Journal of Psychiatric Practice, 27*(1). 33–42.

Greenwood, P. (2016). Moving practice into theory: Bringing real-world considerations to a systemic perspective on incarceration. *Couple and Family Psychology: Research and Practice, 5*(2), 105-108. https://doi-org/10.1037/cfp0000061

Johnson, R. C. (2009). Ever-increasing levels of parental incarceration and the consequences for children. In S. Raphael & M. Stoll (Eds.), *Do prisons make us safer? The benefits and costs of the prison boom* (pp. 177–206). New York: Russell Sage Foundation

Johnson, E. I., & Easterling, B. (2012). Understanding unique effects of parental incarceration on children: Challenges, progress, and recommendations. *Journal of Marriage and Family, 74*(2), 342–356. https://doi.org/10.1111/j.1741-3737.2012.00957.x

Kajeepeta, S., Mauro, P. M., Keyes K. M., El-Sayed, A. M., Rutherford, C. G., & Prins, S. J. (2021). Association between county jail incarceration and cause-specific county mortality in the USA,1987–2017: A retrospective, longitudinal study. *The Lancet Public Health, 6*(4), 240–248.

Kazura, K. (2018). Relationship intervention for inmates and their partners: Bringing couples together before release. *International Journal of Offender Therapy and Comparative Criminology, 62*(9). https://doi.org/10.1177/0306624X17721525

Lemert, E. M. (1974). Beyond mead: The societal reaction to deviance. *Social Problems, 21*, 457–468.

Levin, A. (2019). History of patient advocacy in psychiatry: From passive patient to active participant. *Psychiatric News, 54*(17). https://doi.org/10.1176/appi.pn.2019.9a17

Link, B. G., & Phelan, J. C. (2001). Conceptualizing stigma. *Annual Review of Sociology, 27*, 400–423.

Lurigio, A. J. (2011). People with serious mental illness in the criminal justice system: Causes, consequences, and correctives. *Prison Journal, 91*(3_suppl), 66S–86S.

Major, B., & Sawyer, P. J. (2009). Attributions to discrimination: Antecedents and consequences. In T. D. Nelson (Ed.), *Handbook of prejudice, stereotyping, and discrimination* (pp. 89–110). New York: Psychology Press.

Morenoff, J. D., & Harding, D. J. (2014). Incarceration, prisoner reentry, and communities. *Annual Review of Sociology, 40*(1), 411–421. https://doi.org/10.1146/annurev-soc-071811-145511.

Murphey, D., & Cooper, P. M. (2015). Parents behind bars: What happens to their children? *Child Trends*. https://cms.childtrends.org/wp-content/uploads/2015/10/2015-42ParentsBehindBars.pdf

Poehlmann, J. (2005). Representations of attachment relationships in children of incarcerated mothers. *Child Development, 76*, 679–696. https://doi.org/10.1111/j.1467-8624.2005.00871.x

Poehlmann, J., Dallaire, D. H., Loper, A. B., & Shear, L. D. (2010). Children's contact with their incarcerated parents: Research findings and recommendations. *American Psychologist, 65*(6), 575–598. https://doi.org/10.1037/a0020279

Rose, D. R., & Clear, T. R. (1998). Incarceration, social capital, and crime: Implications for social disorganization. *Criminology, 36*, 441–479.

Saha, G. (2021). Advocacy in mental health. *Indian Journal of Psychiatry, 63*(6), 523–526. https://doi.org/10.4103/indianjpsychiatry.indianjpsychiatry_901_21

Sexton, T. L. (2016). Incarceration as a family affair: Thinking beyond the individual. *Couple and Family Psychology: Research and Practice, 5*(2), 61–64. https://dx. doi.org/10.1037/cfp0000062

Shlafer, R. J., & Poehlmann, J. (2010). Attachment and caregiving relationships in families affected by parental incarceration. *Attachment & Human Development, 12*, 395–415.

Tadros, E., Dignam, C., & Welshans, E. (2024). We are all sentenced: The lived experience of mothers with an adult incarcerated daughter. *Feminist Criminology*. https://doi.org/10.1177/15570851241260912.

Tadros, E., Hutcherson, R., & Aguirre, N. (2023). How is family therapy discussed in the literature on incarceration? A systematic review. *The American Journal of Family Therapy, 51*(5), 673–691. https://doi.org/10.1080/01926187.2022.2031343

Tadros, E., Presley, S., & Gomez, E (2022). "Not for the weak": The lived experiences of women in romantic relationships with incarcerated individuals. *Crime & Delinquency, 68*(2). https://doi.org/10.1177/00111287221077657.

Tadros, E., Presley, S., & Gomez, E. (2025). "Who are you really punishing?" Mothers' experiences with an incarcerated son. *Crime & Delinquency, 71*(4), 1210–1239. https://doi.org/10.1177/00111287221146544.

Thomas, K. C., Ellis, A. R., Konrad, T. R., Holzer, C. E., & Morrissey, J. P. (2009). County-level estimates of mental health professional shortage in the United States. *Psychiatric Services, 60*(10), 1323–1328. https://doi.org/10.1176/ps.2009.60.10.1323.

Thompson, R. A. (2008). Early attachment and later development: Familiar questions, new answers. In J. Cassidy & P. R. Shaver (Eds.), *Handbook of attachment: Theory, research, and clinical applications* (2nd ed., pp. 348–365). New York: Guilford Press.

Travis, J., Solomon, A. L., & Waul, M. (2001). *From prison to home: dimensions and consequences of prisoner reentry.* Washington, DC: The Urban Institute.

United States Commission on Civil Rights (2019). *Collateral consequences: The crossroads of punishment, redemption, and the effects of communities.* Washington, DC: Author.

Wacquant, L. (2009). *Punishing the poor: The neoliberal government of social insecurity.* Durham, NC: Duke University Press. https://doi.org/10.1215/9780822392255.

Wakefield, S., & Wildeman, C. (2014). *Children of the prison boom: Mass incarceration and the future of American inequality.* Oxford: Oxford University Press.

Winnick, T. A., & Bodkin, M. (2008). Anticipated stigma and stigma management among those to be labeled "Ex-con". *Deviant Behavior, 29*, 295–333.

Index

For Product Safety Concerns and Information please contact our EU representative GPSR@taylorandfrancis.com
Taylor & Francis Verlag GmbH, Kaufingerstraße 24, 80331 München, Germany

www.ingramcontent.com/pod-product-compliance
Ingram Content Group UK Ltd.
Pitfield, Milton Keynes, MK11 3LW, UK
UKHW022352190926
475702UK00015B/2251
* 9 7 8 1 0 3 2 8 8 2 2 5 3 *

PARANORMAL AND ANOMALOUS EXPERIENCES IN THERAPY

This groundbreaking book gives counselors, psychologists, social workers, clergy, and other helping professionals the tools they need to ethically and compassionately support clients who report paranormal or anomalous experiences. Without debating the reality of ghosts, visions, or unexplained encounters, Dr. Steve F. Bain and Dr. Kristopher K. Garza focus on what truly matters—the emotional and psychological impact such experiences can have on a person's life. This book offers strategies for bracketing personal beliefs, fostering empathy, and guiding clients toward meaning and peace. For the first time, mental health professionals are provided with a concise, accessible resource that bridges the gap between clinical training and the lived realities of those who face the mysterious. This readable, practical book is the definitive resource for introducing compassionate skills that you as a professional can implement in your sessions.

Key features include:

Multicultural Approach: Understand how culture affects work with clients dealing with unexplained phenomena.

Theoretical Foundations: Learn from time-honored theoretical perspectives that provide a basis for assisting clients with perception, awareness, acceptance, and personal growth.

Ethical Considerations: Examine ethical obligations to practice and model non-maleficence, beneficence, and veracity when working with clients reporting unexplained phenomena.

G.H.O.S.T. Method: Explore and integrate basic counseling skills while applying the G.H.O.S.T. method when addressing paranormal experiences.

God and Ghosts: Discover how to reconcile paranormal experiences with the spirituality and beliefs of your clients—as well as your own.

Evidence-Based Strategies: Review proven treatment approaches designed to strengthen your therapeutic toolbox.

Case Studies, Examples, and Exercises: Field-based stories and exercises designed to help you read, reflect, analyze, and integrate key concepts.

Accepting the Paranormal as Normal: Develop a genuine, empathetic approach toward clients that does not compromise your own beliefs.

Steve F. Bain is a counseling professor with over forty years of pastoral and professional experience. His research explores rural mental health, trauma, and integration of paranormal phenomena in counseling.

Kristopher K. Garza is a counseling professor and counseling supervisor whose work focuses on rural mental health, ethics, anxiety, and supporting clients processing paranormal experiences through meaningful, culturally sensitive counseling.